http://therapist2013.wix.com/e-therapy

Dedicated to my Loving Sister, Shirley A. Carlisle

Who supported all of my educational endeavors

INTRODUCTION

What is normal? Everyone struggles with the word "normal." Who's to say what is normal or who is not normal. If you ask each individual the question, what does normal mean to them, you will get a different answer every time. There are many descriptions for what people call "normal." There's not one person on this planet that's the same. We are all unique individuals. Normal is defined by behavioral experts, as behavior that is normal for an individual when it is consistent with the most common behavior for that person. "Normal is also used to describe when someone's behavior conforms to the most common behavior in society." Definitions of normality can vary by person, time, place, and situation. "It changes along with changing society standards and norms." It's been said "to describe normal as being behavior often recognized in contrast to abnormality." In its simplest form, "normality is seen as good while abnormality is seen as bad." "Someone being seen as "normal" or "not normal" can have social ramifications, such as being included, excluded or stigmatized by larger society."

This mental health coping skills book will offer a cumulative of technique from months of research and feedback from a diverse group of individuals with mental health disorders. Although some of the technique can be found, and used differently for several mental health disorders, the coping techniques were gather together to be conveniently found in one book. This book will show you how to turn technique into coping skills and choose the best skills for each mental illness as well as, help you make the right choices when selecting alternative holistic ways to treat your mental illness. Each technique in this book was tested and found to be most helpful in helping individuals living with a mental health diagnosis live a "normal" life. It's been said that coping skill techniques is essential in maintaining control over any mental health condition. What works for one person may not work for another, and no one treatment is appropriate in all cases. Just as the symptoms and causes of mental illness are different in different people, so are the ways to feel better.

It is suggested to use these coping techniques accompanied with other treatments such as therapy (http://therapist2013.wix.com/e-therapy) and medication, or the techniques can be done alone. There is evidence showing individuals who need and use coping skills are growing at an alarming rate. However, I am not trying to reinvent the wheel; I believe this book will clearly give examples of coping techniques that will fit your mental health needs. The easy-to-do techniques will enable you to learn the technique in a short period of time, and it can be done anywhere. In many cases, you may find that alternating or combining different techniques will help you stay motivated and provide you with the best results. The secret to success is to follow the techniques until you find the one that works for you.

Note to the reader: No coping skill technique replaces the medical advice of a physician. Please be certain to consult with your doctor before making any decisions that affect your health, particularly if you suffer from any medical condition or have any symptoms that may require treatment. There is always in any process the possibility that someone could experience some discomfort.

http://therapist2013.wix.com/e-therapy

CONTENTS

- **Medication for Mental Health Disorders   1-2**
- **Diet and Mental Health   3-4**
- **Juicing and Mental Illness   5-6**
- **Vitamin Therapy for Mental Health Disorders   7-8**
- **Nutritional Therapy   9-10**
- **Herbal Alternatives for Mental Health   11-15**

CHAPTER: (1) ANXIETY DISORDER   16-17

- Breathing Exercise   18-19
- Ice Water   20-21
- Meditation   22-23
- Stay Busy   24-25
- Moderate Exercise   26-27
- Prayer   28-29
- Social Support   30-31
- Clear You're Thoughts   32-33
- Stay Sober   34-35
- Journaling and Anxiety   36-37
- Music and Anxiety   38-39
- Hot Shower   40-41
- Bike Riding   42-43
- Do something for yourself   44-45
- Get Motivated and Think Positive   64-47
- Higher Power   48-49
- Relaxation   50-51

CHAPTER: (2) MANAGING DEPRESSION   52-53

- Talk about it   54-55
- Seek understanding   56-57
- List Solutions   58-59

- Hotline   60-61
- Watch Television   62-63
- Read   64-65
- Music and Depression   66-67
- Journaling and Depression   68-69
- Gratitude List   70-71
- Crafts   72-73
- Challenge Negative Thinking   74-75
- Take a Break   76-77
- Exercise and Depression   78-79
- Healthy Self-Esteem   80-81
- Don't Worry be Happy   82-83
- Talk with Counselor/Case Manager   84-85

CHAPTER: (3) AUDITORY HALLUCINATIONS   86-87

- Distractions   88-89
- Earplugs   90-91
- Thinking (cognitive Approach)   92-93
- Concentration   94-95
- Relaxation   96-97
- Talking   98-99
- Remind yourself it's not real   100-101
- Talk to other Voice Hearers   102-103
- Focusing   104-105
- Medication   106-107

CHAPTER: (4) DRUGS AND ALCOHOL   109-109

- Alcohol Use and Abuse: What you should know 110-111
- Attend Alcoholic Anonymous (AA)   112-113
- Detoxification Program   114-115
- Remove Drug Paraphernalia   116-117

- Replacing Addictions with a Healthy Obsessions   118-119
- Prayer   120-121
- Big Book (AA)   122-123
- Sponsor   124-125
- Building a Recovery Support Group   126-127
- People, Places, and Things   128-129

CHAPTER: (5) STRESS MANAGEMENT   130-131

- Cleaning   132-133
- Talking   134-135
- Massage Therapy   136-137
- Venting   138-139
- Build Relationship   140-141
- YOGA   142-143
- Acupuncture   144-145
- Ask for Help   146-147
- Read   148-149
- Stress Balls   150-151
- Take a Nap   152-153
- Arts and Craft   154-155
- Stress Relief Games   156-157
- Prioritize   158-159
- Pray/Church   160-161
- Walking to Relieve Stress   162-163

CHAPTER (6): ANGER MANAGEMENT   164-165

- Tools for Anger Management   166-167
- Anger Support Hotline   168-169
- Music Therapy   170-171
- Understanding/Compassion   172-173
- Remove Yourself   174-175

- Triggers and Distractions — 176-177
- Emotional Control — 178-179
- Breathing Techniques — 180-181
- Laugh — 182-183
- Journaling and Anger — 184-185
- Reactions vs. Response — 186-187
- Assertive — 188-189
- Expectations — 190-191
- Don't Stuff Anger — 192-193
- Don't Attack or Blame others — 194-195
- Have your Support point it out — 196-197

CHAPTER (7): MOOD SWINGS — 198-199

- Talk About It — 200-201
- Take a Break and Sit Quietly — 202-203
- Be Consequence Aware — 204-205
- Positive Self-Talk — 206-207
- Healthy Sleeping Habits — 208-209
- Nutrition — 210-211
- Changing your Perspective — 212-213
- Shift your Feelings — 214-215

CHAPTER (8): RACING THOUGHTS — 216-217

- Writing — 218-219
- Physical Activity — 220-221
- Clearing you Thoughts — 222-223
- Read — 224-225
- Breaking Thoughts into Smaller Pieces — 226-227
- Developing a Daily List — 228-229
- Support/Group therapy — 230-231
- Focus — 232-233
- Progressive Muscle Relaxation — 234-235

- Shut off your Brain before Bed Time   236-237

CHAPTER (9): OBESSIVE HOUGHTS/BEHAVIORS 238-239

- Talk to your Doctor   240-241
- Humor   242-243
- Peggy Back Reality/Reality Testing   244-245
- Reactive Distraction/Proactive Distraction   246-247
- Visualization/Guided Imagery Therapy   248-249
- Meditation   250-251
- Self-Soothing Activity   252-253
- Pros and Cons for (OCD)   254-255
- Observe your Behavior   256-257

CHAPTER (10): BOUNDARIES AND LIMITS   258-259

- Operate from Intellectually, Emotionally, and Intuitively   260-261
- Keep your Distance   262-263
- Saying "NO"   264-265
- Be Firm   266-267
- Be Assertive   268-269
- Be Specific   270-271
- Don't be a Doormat   272-273
- Body Language   274-275

CHAPTER (11): ASSERTIVENESS   276-277

- Aggressive   278-279
- Stay Calm Confident and Boost Self-Esteem   280-281
- Be Concise and to the Point   282-283
- Assertive Communication   284-285
- 4 Ideas to Assertiveness   286-287

CHAPTER (12): SUICIDAL IDEATION   288-289

- Call Someone   290-291
- Don't Entertain the Thoughts   292-293
- Distraction   294-295
- Go to a Place where you Feel Safe   296-297
- Keep Medication Locked in a Safe Place   298-299
- Positive Self-Talk/Journal   300-301
- Avoid Drugs and Alcohol   302-303
- Be Mindful   304-305
- Remain Curious   306-307
- Be Safe   308-309
- How to Reduce the Risks   310-311
- Give yourself Small Goals   312-313

CHAPTER (13): COMMUNICATION   314-315

- Long Distance Communication   316-317
- Letter   318-319
- Body Language   320-321
- Non-Verbal Communication Roles   322-323
- Communication Through Touch   324-325
- Humor for Communication and Persuasion   326-327
- Listen   328-329
- Keep Voice Even   330-331
- Proper Language   332-333
- Communicate with love   334-335
- Keep Physical Intimacy Alive   336-337
- Expressing Feelings   338-339
- Agree to Disagree   340-341

CHAPTER (14): FLASHBACKS 341-342

- Write down the Memory 343-344
- Ground Yourself 345-346
- Grounding Techniques 347-348
- Mindfulness 349-350
- Know your Triggers 351-352
- Identify early Warning Signs 353-354
- Us all your Senses 355-356
- Self-Talk 357-358
- Dispute Negative Thoughts 359-360
- People in History and Modern Times who Achieved Great Things 361-366
- Juice Recipes for a Healthier Mental Health 367-374
- Herbal tea for mental health recovery 375-378
- Resources 379-381
- Message from the Author 382-383

MEDICATION FOR MENTAL HEALTH DISORDERS

Studies have shown, people who take prescribed medication for mental illness complain about side effects from the medication. It's been said by my clients "it's like exchanging one mental illness for another." Often, the side effects are the main reason most people stop taking medication. In general, most people would rather deal with the mental illness because the side effects cannot be tolerated. In some cases, individuals were prescribed the maximum dosage that is allowed for a particular medication (under doctor's supervision) and still did not get the relief needed to live a "normal" life. Also, some people may have a few side effects and others have none at all from their medication and on the other hand, other individuals taking the same medication may have a lot of side effects says the Mental Health Foundation. Your reaction to medication depends on many factors, including but not limited to your age, weight, sex, metabolic rate, and other medicines you might be taking.

Secondly, for some people, "drugs are a short-term solution used to get them over an immediate crisis." For other people, "drugs are an ongoing, long-term treatment that enables them to live with severe mental health problems." Many people tell me they do not want to stay on medication for years, but it's been said, medication can help stop relapses and re-admissions to hospitals. Doctors also vary in how often they prescribe it, and in what doses. According to the Mental Health Foundation, "all kinds of medication have some placebo (a substance containing no medication) effect and some drug trials have found only light differences between the effects of placebos and active drugs."

Also, it's been said that medication is easier to administer than talking therapies or learning coping skill technique which are also effective for many mental health problems. Most medication has side effects, and some people may have problems when they stop taking the medication as well. Experts believe, for some people side effects can be temporary, and will improve over time as your body adjusts to the medication. However, some side effects can be long lasting and even permanent.

Lastly, researchers have documented, the newer medications that are being developed now tend to have fewer and less harsh side effects for some people says the Mental Health Foundation. Once you begin your medication the symptoms resolve for some people and you are able to get back to your "normal" state of functioning. There is evidence showing, the more "serious side effects are associated with the older antipsychotic medications, such as, Haldol, Stelazine and Thorazine." Most doctors suggest that all of the psychotropic drugs need to reach a therapeutic level before you can see positive results and each psychotropic drug have different length of time to reach their level. This is why I tell my clients it is so important to stay with the prescribed dose and time frame, but this has been an on-going issue for most people and that's way many people never get the therapeutic help needed. If you are having side effects, call your doctor or therapist as soon as possible. Your doctor will help you measure how serious the side effects are and what you can do about them. It is up to you to decide what side effects you can tolerate and what risk you are willing to take.

HOLISTIC MEASURES

DIET AND MENTAL HEALTH

The facts show, in the countries bordering the Mediterranean Sea, diet has always been link to good health and has been associated in reducing the risk of death from heart disease and cancer, as well as a reduced incidence of Parkinson's and Alzheimer's diseases says Mayo Clinic. Similarly, in the last few years scientific studies are starting to give more attention to the effects of diet and our mental health. Diet and mental health are rapidly being linked together as more studies are being made. A detailed report, Feeding Minds from the Mental Health Foundation (MHF) suggests that many Mental Health conditions such as Depression, Schizophrenia, Alzheimer's disease and Attention Deficit Hyperactivity Disorder (ADHD) can be prevented/ treated by consuming the right kinds of food and drinks. Research shows the number of cases of mental illness has been steadily growing and this affects us both socially and economically. The Feeding Minds report suggests that the changes in our diets are contributing factor to this. Dr. Andrew McCulloch from the MHF states that "we are only just beginning to understand how the brain as an organ is influenced by the nutrients it derives from the foods we eat and how diets have an impact on our mental health."

In addition, history tells us for many years the normal treatment for mental health problems has been focused on prescribing drugs to fight the effects of the mental health condition. These drugs such as anti-depressants don't just affect the brain they are supposed to target, the medication also has severe side effects on the behavior of the user.

This is why I have heard people on anti-depressants often report feeling like 'zombies' and not feeling like their true selves because the drugs fog their "normal" thought patterns. If in fact eating the right diet and consuming the right foods, drinks and supplements can help prevent mental health problems then the promotion of these possibilities are of great importance thus the reason for this book. Researchers have documented Mental Health prevention is better than the cure as the benefits include but not limited to:

1. Prevention of emotional distress for the individual and their friends/family
2. Reduced pharmaceutical bills
3. No negative physical/emotional side effects that can be associated with prescribed drugs (medication).
4. Benefits to physical well being as the individual will be consuming a well balanced diet so risk of obesity, heart conditions etc. is less.
5. Reduction of hospital admittance

JUICING AND MENTAL ILLNESS

It's been said when you are diagnosed with Depression, Anxiety or a Mental Illness, or know someone who suffers from this, it can be a very difficult time. However, you can also look at it as an opportunity to learn about juicing and its healing power. Research has shown natural approaches to treating Depression and Mental Illness have been proven to work over a long period of time in compared to the conventional approach. Whether you are already taking anti-depressant medication or are considering alternative treatment, I believe if you are equipped with the proper information you will be able to make well informed decision for your mental health. In researching, I found the documentary for 'Food Matters'. The documentary pointed out countless resources and lifestyles considerations that is consider important in your mission to healing. If you haven't seen the DVD it is suggested that you view it to help you discover more about the world of juicing.

In addition, The Natural News suggest juicing is far more than just a health fad, juicing raw fruits and vegetables every day continues to be one of the best ways to obtain fresh, bio-available nutrients in therapeutic, health-transforming doses. The short-term health benefits of juicing include things like increased energy levels and digestive relief, while the long-term health benefits include chronic illness prevention that could add both life to your years and years to your life. Experts believe these are two specific ways that juicing can help as related to mental illness.

Improve mood. Mental illness is becoming more common in today's world, and often unrecognized, the cause of this may be simple nutrient deficiency. If not addressed, mental illnesses cause by nutrient deficiency can take a serious toll on physical health, which is why it is important to correct it early through juicing and other nutritional means.

To add, "Vitamins act as catalytic agents in the body, helping to speed up the chemical processes vital for both survival and brain function," explains Dr. Hyla Cass. Dr. Hyla Cass states the importance of nutrition in maintaining a healthy mental state "As a result, vitamin deficiencies can sometimes manifest themselves as depression. Fortunately, when these deficiencies are treated with supplements or juicing, there is a reversal in symptoms."

Correct nutrient deficiencies. It has been said, many chronic and mental illnesses are a direct result of nutrient deficiencies, which can be easily and quickly remedied through juicing. Since they provide an easily-digestible source of a mass of vitamins, minerals and other nutrients, fresh juices are one of the simplest ways to avoid developing heart disease, organ failure, cancer, mental illness, and various other health conditions that can result in early death.

VITAMIN THERAPY FOR MENTAL HEALTH DISORDERS

Nutritional Therapy:

According to Leonard John Hoffer, people who suffer from mental illness such as depression, anxiety, bipolar disorder, schizophrenia, etc., may not think a physical problem could be part of the cause. The facts show people who have vitamin deficiencies often experience mental health problems and/or are diagnosed with a mental illness.

Here is a list of vitamins that Hoffer suggested that helps with most mental health disorders.

Vitamin C Deficiency: It's been said most people associate vitamin C with helping to prevent colds and flu, also, those with a severe deficiency of this vitamin may experience symptoms of mental illness including: depression, confusion, insomnia, and anxiety. According to Dr. Leonard John Hoffer, author of "Vitamin Therapy in Schizophrenia", schizophrenic patients have a tendency to be deficient in this critical vitamin, due to poor diet. It is recommended that up to 6 grams of vitamin C can be taken to reduce schizophrenic symptoms.

Vitamin D Deficiency: According to experts, this vitamin is called 'the sunshine vitamin' because we absorb this vitamin directly through our skin when we step outside. Unfortunately, because of increasing incidents of skin cancer, vitamin D deficiency is the most common vitamin deficiency on record. It can cause mental illness symptoms such as: "Seasonal affective disorder, depression, irritability, psychosis."

According to a New York study done on teenagers admitted to the emergency room for psychotic symptoms, over 40 percent with symptoms of psychosis were deficient in vitamin D.

Omega 3 Deficiency: Research shows Omega 3 is an essential fatty acid and the body cannot produce it on its own. Study has shown Omega 3 can be absorbed through supplemental sources and it is critical for good neurological health, and a deficiency in it has been linked to mental illness symptoms such as: depression, mood disorders, ADHD, and behavioral problems in children.

Magnesium Deficiency: Researchers have documented this trace mineral is responsible for the regulation of over three hundred different functions in the body and a deficiency in it can cause a host of troubling mental symptoms such as: sever anxiety, insomnia, irritability, confusion, ADHD, and sensitivity to light and sound. "Magnesium deficiency is also noted to cause physical symptoms such as twitching, trembling, muscle cramping, muscle weakness and allergies." Those who feel they do not get enough of the magnesium they need from solid food may benefit from juicing or supplements to calm symptoms and help the nervous system heal and repair itself.

NUTRITIONAL THERAPY:

Vitamin B12 Deficiency: "Those who have difficulty absorbing nutrients from food due to celiac disease, crohn's disease, intestinal surgery where part of the intestine was removed and other mal-absorption problems may suffer from vitamin B12 (folic acid) deficiency." "This vitamin deficiency can cause severe symptoms of mental illness including: moodiness, mania, hallucinations, psychosis, paranoia, insomnia, and learning difficulties says Hoffer.

    In conclusion, anyone suffering from mental illness and unable to continue taking medication because of side effects or want to add this to their wellness regiment should continue the therapy and medication they are on and inform their doctor or therapist that they are interested in nutrition treatments. If you suddenly stop psychiatric medication it may cause damaging side effects. Tapering off medication should be done gradually and under a doctor's supervision. Mental illness can make everyday life difficult. Treating these symptoms using nutritional therapy may be just what you need to get back on tract to wellness. "If you find the doctor currently treating your mental illness not open to nutritional therapy, continue with your treatment and make an appointment with a more open-minded physician or naturopath who can help make your transition a little easier" Says Hoffer.

    In the end it might surprise most people that taking vitamins for your mental health can be one of the most effective natural treatments. "Vitamins play key roles in the chemical reactions that occur within our bodies" says Hoffer.

Also, vitamins play a vital role in our metabolism and brain function. "If the right amounts of vitamin are not present, our bodies cannot function correctly and often cause anxiety or depression." To find out if you have a vitamin deficiencies ask your doctor to schedule you for testing.

Minister about the shortcomings of your life and you will not only heal others you will heal yourself."
--Stephanie Lee—

HERBAL ALTERNATIVES FOR MENTAL HEALTH

According to Gayle Eversole, DHom, PhD, RN (CP), a medical herbalist, more and more attention is on the use of herbs in the treatment of mental and emotional difficulties. She states the most well known herb now, is Saint John's Wort. One study reported in the Pharmer's Almanac (Herb Pharm), showed that the bioflavonoid compounds in Saint John's Wort (SJW) are required for effectiveness. "Standardize SJW compounds eliminate the bioflavonoid compounds eliminate the bioflavonoid compounds." This finding supports how importance it is to use whole herb remedies.

She goes on to say teas and other water based extraction methods, or the newer extraction processes with grain alcohol, with or without water, are the most effective methods to administer herbs. Often, standardize compounds that manufactured the parts of herbs used may not be the specific part known to have medicinal impact. "Trends in the herbal market place lead to many products made by manufactures with little or no knowledge of herbal compounding and preparation."

Unfortunately, politics and pharmaceutical interests also have a major effect on the quality and availability of effective herbal products, and cost. One example of this is a chain of products made by a well-known drug company. Looking for profit than the understanding of "herbs and healers", this product line (vitamins mixed and herbs) is promoted as the only products to use for results. "This same company was cited in a recent claim of price fixing in the vitamin market." The drug company products were also found to be at least 50 percent more expensive than products made by herbal companies says doctor Eversole.

Herb	Nutrients
Hops	B complex, magnesium, zinc, copper, iodine, manganese, iron, sodium,
Oat straw	Silicon, calcium, phosphorus, vitamins A, B1, B2, E
Scullcap	Calcium, potassium, magnesium, iron, zinc, vitamins C, E,
Valerian	Magnesium, potassium, copper, zinc
Wood Betony	Magnesium, manganese, phosphorus

Take a look at the chart Dr. Eversole provided below that shows several herbs used for mental health, and some of the nutrients they contain:

According to Eversole, most people are familiar with SJW and valerian. "These herbs are classified as a nervine-sedative because of the primary way in which they work on the brain and nervous system."

Also, Eversole, talks about SJW describing its "star shaped yellow flower
Beautiful enough to make anyone with the blues feel happier." SJW has been shown to be effect for anxiety, depression, sleep, and headache. It can be helpful in hysteria and brain fog. It also has MAO inhibitor qualities [MAO=Monoamine oxidize, an enzyme that functions in the nervous system], and offers a lot of benefit in the treatment of pain, including phantom pain, and as an anti-viral.

It's been said some use Valerian root as a muscle relaxant and to help with sleep. It embodies volatile oils and alkaloids that create a calming, sedative effect. It is a great muscle relaxant, pain reliever, and helps with nervous tension. It is not recommended for children, but it has been used in compounds for children with severe agitation and "ADHD." If experiencing a paradoxical effect with valerian, it has been suggest replacing with Scullcap. Scullcap is said to be like quinine as a nerve stimulant without any side effects. Historically it is called the food of the nerves, offering almost immediate relief from all acute and chronic nerve afflictions and weakness. The benefits of this herb were noted in the 1600's. It is said to be a good herb for children, for people with seizures, Parkinson's disease, neuralgia, St. Vitus dance, and spinal meningitis.

In addition, another herb people talk about is Passionflower. Passionflower is known as most people favorite remedies. There is a lot of evidence showing it being used specifically to help people withdraw from prescription anti-depressants and sleeping medication. It is shown to be good for children, and in many European countries is the treatment of choice for Add/ADHD. Also, research has shown it to be good for agitation and it is recommended for elderly persons who are institutionalized, as an alternative to Haldol. It's been said to be a good choice for insomnia, children with convulsions, and headache. Passionflower, according to J Clin Pharm Therapy, is equally effective as often prescribed anti-anxiety agents, with no side effects.

Lastly, a rare herb used in cases for anxiety related gastric symptoms, is Lady's Slipper Orchild. Experts would not suggest common use of Lady's Slipper because it is almost extinct in the wild. However, it is said to be the safest know nervine in the plant kingdom, and the best.

It is very slow acting, yet it is healing to all parts of the nervous system. It works mainly on the medulla to regulate breathing, sweating, saliva, and heart function. It contains a high level of all B complex vitamins. This is a good herb for complete nervous exhaustion and chores. Kava in the right form is an excellent herb, but at this time its use is being questioned, and access is limited.

Examples of herbs selected by a clinical herbalist in place of common prescription medicines:

Neurotransmitter	Common diagnosis	Rx	Herb
GABA	Anxiety	Benzodiazepines	Valerian, Hops
Norepinephrine	Anxiety, sleep disorder, depression, ADD	Tri-cyclics, Ritalin	St. John's Wort
Serotonin	Depression, anxiety	SSRIs	St. John's Wort
Beta endorphins	Mood, sleep, and pain dis-orders	Opiate narcotics	SJW, California Poppy, Kava, Nutmeg, Borage, Lotus oil

> Excerpted from an article by David Overton, PA-C, The Herbalist, 1997.

Other herbs to consider are California Poppy, Hops (good for making a "sleep pillow" to tuck in your pillow case), Feverfew, Chamomile (avoid if you have a ragweed allergy), Catnip, Licorice (use with caution with hypertension), Ginseng, Blue Virvian, Blue Cohosh, Skunk Cabbage, Clove, Cyani, Evening Primrose oil, Fennel (a sedative for children), Gentian (eating dis-orders), Ginkgo, Gotu Kola, Lobelia, Rosemary, Suma (mood swings), Wild Lettuce, Wild Cherry (feeds the pituitary and pineal glands).

It is said when combining herbs for emotional treatments, look to herbs for liver and gall bladder function, and to those with hormonal balancing properties. For those unfamiliar with the therapeutic use of herbs, it is best to work with and experienced herbal practitioner. Often you will be able to find a clinical herbalist who will work in conjunction with your physician.

Chapter 1

ANXIETY DISORDER

According to the American Psychiatric Association: Diagnostic and Statistical Manual of Mental Disorders, there are several recognized types of anxiety disorders which include:

Panic disorder: People with this condition have feelings of terror that strike suddenly and repeatedly with no warning. Other symptoms of a panic attack include sweating, chest pain, palpitations, and a feeling of choking, which may make the person feel like he or she is having a heart attack or "going crazy". DSM

Obsessive-compulsive disorder (OCD): People with OCD are plagued by constant thoughts of fears that cause them to perform certain rituals or routines. The disturbing thoughts are called obsessions, and the rituals are called compulsions. DSM

Post-traumatic stress disorder (PTSD): PTSD is a condition that can develop following a traumatic and/or terrifying event. People with PTSD often have lasting and frightening thoughts and memories of the event and tend to be emotionally numb. DSM

Social anxiety disorder: Also called social phobia, social anxiety disorder involves overwhelming worry and self-consciousness about everyday social situations. The worry often centers on a fear of being judged by others, or behaving in a way that might cause embarrassment or lead to ridicule. DSM

Specific phobias: A specific phobia is an intense fear of a specific object or situation, such as snakes, heights, or flying. DSM

Generalized anxiety disorder: This disorder involves excessive, unrealistic worry and tension, even if there is little or nothing to provoke and anxiety. DSM

*Symptoms of an Anxiety Disorder: Feeling of panic, fear, and uneasiness, uncontrollable, obsessive thoughts, repeated thoughts or flashbacks of traumatic experiences, nightmares, ritualistic behaviors, such as repeated hand washing, problems sleeping, cold or sweaty hands and/or feet, shortness of breath, palpitations, an inability to be still and calm, dry mouth, numbness or tingling in the hands or feet, nausea, muscle tension, and dizziness. DSM

BREATHING EXERCISE

It's very important to know and understand how breathing can help with our mind, body, and soul. It's been said by physical fitness experts, breathing exercises are good for anxiety because it's fast, free, simple, and you can do them almost anywhere and at anytime. Here are three techniques that are commonly used for quick anxiety relief.

Basic Breathing exercise:

1. Sit or stand in a relaxed position. Slowly inhale through your nose, counting to five in your head. Let the air out from your month, counting to eight in your head as it leaves your lungs. Repeat

Belly Breath exercise:

This is an exercise for learning to breathe abdominally comes from the University of Missouri, Kansas City Extension Center. Lie flat on your back to get the right sense of deep breathing. Place your hands, palms down, on your stomach, at the base of the rib cage. Make sure that the middle fingers of both hands are barely touching each other, and take a deep breath. Exhale, and begin again. For best results, practice this exercise for five minutes.

Guided Visualization with Breathing:

It's been established that both visualization and breathing exercises is great anxiety relief strategies. This is how it's done. Head straight for your "happy place," no question asked. You can find your happy place with a coach, therapist or helpful relaxation recording as your guide. Breathe deeply while focusing on pleasant, positive images to replace any negative thoughts.

Psychologist Dr. Ellen Langer explains that while it's just one means of achieving mindfulness, "Guided visualization helps put you in the place you want to be, rather than letting your mind go to the internal conversation that is stressful."

"Breathing optimally is a primary key to longevity. You can regain a lot of what you lost or improve most of what you have."

--Michael Grant White—

ICE WATER

It's been suggested by my clients when they dip their face in cold water, take a cold baths, or cold shower it help to relieve their anxiety. According to Steve Mensing, (Arthur of Emoclear Self-Helpapedia: Powerful Techniques to Optimize Your Emotions, Beliefs, and Behaviors) this is known as water therapy and here's how it's done. He suggested you slowly introduce your body to cold water by starting with warm then turning the water to the cold temperature this will give your body time to adjust to it. After awhile you will get use to it. Some feel it is a stimulating experience and it wakes you up. The technical name for applying cold water to your face is called Dive Reflex. The expert says the Dive Reflex, originated from cold water diving. It is said to be a first rate nerve stimulation method capable of chilling down or lowering anxiety, panic, stress and body-wide inflammation as well as elevating moods quickly.

The Two Basic Steps Mensing Recommends for Using the Drive Reflex:

1. Fill a small plastic bag full of ice or ice cubes and wait until the outside of the bag is cold. If you are very sensitive to cold, you can wrap the bag in a thin cotton cloth or towel. Fill your mouth with saliva, and fully submerge your tongue for the remainder of the Dive Reflex. Either imagine a lemon slice in your mouth or use a real one to help you salivate. Or you can take a sip of lukewarm water and keep it there for the remainder of the exercise. It will also stimulate the nerve.

2. For 30 seconds to 1 minute press the ice bag to your face from your scalp line to your lips. Your skin, making contact with the bag, will feel some pleasant numbness.

After 30 to 60 seconds remove the bag and put it back in a freezer or cooler. You will begin to feel mildly upbeat. Within minutes your anxiety and tension will begin to evaporate until it vanishes. Depending on each individual the anti-anxiety affects should last from 40 minutes to 90 minutes. The mood elevation should go on from 40 minutes to an hour or so. You can reply the ice bag and perform the Dive Reflex whenever required.

"Mental health needs a great deal of attention. It's the final taboo and it needs to be faced and dealt with."
--Adam Ant--

MEDITATION

According to Elizabeth Scott, Arthur of Stress Management, there are many different ways to experience the benefits of meditation. We will look at how to get the full benefits that will allow us to release tension that causes anxiety. One easy method and commonly used is meditating in the bath. This is one place where most people will go at the end of the day. "A hot bath and meditation combine have the soothing benefits that will relax tired muscles, provide a relaxing atmosphere (add candles), and is said to lower anxiety." If you take time for meditation you get to experience a very peaceful enjoyable time in your day. For me a good meditation can last about an hour, but always make available at lease a minimum of 15 minutes for meditation where you won't be interrupted. For most people, that may means moving your schedule around. For example, set your phone to go straight into your voice mail, telling others family members not to disturb you unless it's an emergency. And, as you run the bath, it is suggested that you incorporate some of the benefits of aromatherapy by using bubble bath or bath oils scented with lavender (for relaxing) peppermint (more alert) or another scent that you really like.

Also, practice belly breathing exercise by allowing your breathing to get slower, and deeper, allow your belly to rise and fall with each breath. It's been said this type of breathing is more natural and can help turn off your stress responses if it was still triggered from earlier in the day. Now add mindfulness by focusing on the sensations you feel in your body. For example, be aware of how warm the water feels on your skin, the pressure of the tub against your back and clear you mind of all other thoughts.

Try to keep your mind quiet and focused only on the present moment. Mindfulness is a process that will bring you to the here and now. It's been said the benefits from meditation is numerous and is more commonly practice. You don't have to become a skilled mediator to gain benefits from meditative practice. In fact, highly anxious people will find that the meditation techniques are easier to follow, and they may wish to choose one of them as a long-term method to relax your muscles and quite your mind.

However, it is the process of practicing meditation that provides the valuable understanding that you can directly apply to controlling panic, even if you only practice the technique for several weeks, it will help.

"Women in particular need to keep an eye on their physical and mental health, because if we're scurrying to and from appointments and errands, we don't have a lot of time to take care of ourselves. We need to do a better job of putting ourselves higher on our own 'to do' list."
--Michelle Obama—

STAY BUSY

Some people reported staying busy is helpful for their anxiety because it helps them to escape for all of their thoughts. There is a lot of evidence that shows when you're alone and quite your thoughts seem to go through you mind, sometimes fast and sometimes slow. Anxiety has a way of controlling your thoughts weather they're negative or positive. Those individuals who have anxiety tend to want to stay home and be alone. It's been said sometimes just being around people can be a challenge. What you should be doing is creating good memories for positive thoughts. According to the Law of Attraction, what you think about you bring about. If you change the way you think to positive thoughts your mood will shift. Start thinking positive thoughts when you get up in the morning until you go to bed at night. Also, it is important that you try to be around people even if it appears to be hard to do, if you do decide to be alone, try working on crossword puzzles, paint, make a phone call or draw a picture. The object is to try to stay busy and do things that will allow you to use your brain. The facts shows when you're busy your mind learns how to cope with anxiety better. Try to avoid ways and places where you are alone with your thoughts.

To illustrate, here are some activities that is suggested to help you stay busy. You can participate in some of your hobbies or find new ones. There are so many things to do and enjoy in the world, such as baking, sports, arts and crafts, collecting, scrap booking, photography or writing, the list is endless. Or you can use your time to learn more and get deeper into the details of you hobbies, and join professional associations related to you hobbies as well.

Also, try to be in the moment while you are at your job or school. Focus on doing your best that day, learning and teaching others, as well as accomplishing your tasks. One present moment will lead to the next, and before you know it the day will be over.

Remember, the key is to stay around positive people because positive people will help motivate you, help you develop and discover you creativity as well as a good companion for traveling. Lastly, doing things at the spur of the moment can be adventurous however, try to make plans for a month it can be helpful to know what you are going to do in the days to come. Make a schedule for the day, week, or month whatever works for you in your life.

"Self-esteem is as important to our well-being as legs are to a table. It is essential for physical and mental health and for happiness."

--Louise Hart--

MODERATE EXERCISE

More and more conscious Americans are getting involved in exercising. We are discovering that exercise is good for our mental, physical and emotional health. And it's been said it's helpful for most people for easing anxiety. "Moderate exercise has been shown to have a significant effect on anxiety and mood," said Marla Deibler, PsyD, a clinical psychologist and director of The Center for Emotional Health of Greater Philadelphia. Research shows, exercise reduces the stress hormones adrenaline and cortisol. And it stimulates the construction of feel-good endorphins. It also leads to an increase in activity levels in the serotonergic system, which may help to decrease anxiety and improve mood. Plus, "moderate to intense exercise raises core body temperature, which is accompanied by a simultaneous reduction in muscle tension, thereby affecting the experience of anxiety. "Whether you struggle with occasional anxiety or a diagnosable disorder, exercise can help." It's a powerful part of your self-care routine and a very effective coping skill for treating anxiety.

In addition, "Exercise is the only thing you can start today that is as powerful as anxiety medication." It has been studied to a great extent, and there is a lot of evidence showing people that exercise regularly actually get as much relief as those taking medicine prescribe for anxiety. "That's because intense long term exercise releases endorphins a neurotransmitter in the brain that is released in order to reduce pain but has the secondary benefits of reducing anxiety" as well. Further, there are other benefits such as, "exercise reduces muscle tension, promotes sleep, and improves self-confidence.

Research shows, there is no better way to reduce anxiety than to start exercising. If you are serious about reducing your anxiety you need to start your exercise routine today. Also, science has provided some evidence that physically active people have lower rates of anxiety than sedentary people. Exercise may improve mental health by helping the brain cope better with stress. In one study, researchers found that those who got regular vigorous exercise were 25 percent less likely to develop anxiety disorder over the next five years.

"I have long recognized a link between fitness and mental health and I think we need to encourage young people to take part in sports and team activities because we know it has such positive results."

--Tipper Gore--

PRAYER

It's been said by most of my client's they look to their higher power when feeling anxious. However, when anxious and fearful thoughts come into your head, it can be very difficult to quiet your mind and connect with your God in prayer. Especially in the middle of a panic attack, the last thing on your mind is getting alone with God, but prayer is said to be very helpful in stopping those confusing and terrifying thoughts. There is a lot of evidence that shows learning how to pray can calm an anxious mind and fill your heart with peace. No matter who or what your higher power, prayer can work for you. Here is a reminder pull from the Bible for those who have no hope in prayer. "Do not be anxious about anything, but in everything by prayer and petition with thanksgiving present your request to God." And the peace of God, which transcends all understanding, will group your hearts and your minds in Christ Jesus" (Philippians 4:6, 7). Experts believe when anxious thoughts over come your mind you should pray to your higher power and as you do, peace which goes beyond all understanding will quiche your heart and mind." It's been said this can transform an anxious mind into peace of mind. To help you develop and connect to your God it is suggested to follow the five steps.

First, you must believe in your God. Second, know that your God hears you. Third, know who you are in your God. Fourth, understand that words carry power. Fifth, build your prayer muscle with practice. It's been said anxiety works on a very primitive level. "It has a physical component which we can counteract by applying a physical remedy." As well as using the right breathing technique to reduce anxiety and stress. The Harvard Health Blog calls it breath control. The technique has certain similarities with prayerful meditation, and when you combine it with faith, it's called "breathing prayer.

For example, try combing breathing and prayer like this: Close your eyes and inhale slowly, imagining pulling the Spirit in so fully that it fills every pore of your body. Make sure your stomach expands; you want to be pregnant with peace. Exhale slowly through your noses. You can pray while you do this, but if you're anxious when you start, you probably won't think of it until after a few breaths, when your head starts to clear.

Repeat while inhaling	**Repeat while exhaling**
Come Holy spirit...	fill my heart
Calling your God name	grant me your peace
Calling you God name	I love you

Given these points, if you practice when you're not in a wild anxiety mold, it will be easier to pray this way when you are. But "breathing prayer" is a good addition to any regular prayer time.

"I'm by no means condemning prescription medicine for mental health. I've seen it save a lot of people's lives."
                                                            --Zach Braf--

SOCIAL SUPPORT

When you are experiencing high anxiety, it's been suggested by my clients to call someone you trust and feel comfortable talking with. As was previously stated in an earlier chapter, surrounding yourself with positive people always helps when it comes to shifting your mood. According to University of Minnesota, "Taking Charge of your Health Wellbeing," having someone that supports you can be a life saver. Sometimes a friend, other people, or family members you can turn to in times of need or crisis can give you a better focus, and positive self-image. Researchers has found, social support enhance the quality of life, extend your life, and provides a defense against adverse life events.

In addition, whether from a trusted group or valued individual, social support has been shown to reduce the psychological and physiological consequences of stress, and many enhance immune function. Social support is now proven to be a literal life-saver. People that are supported by closer relationships with friend, family, or fellow members of church, or other support groups are less vulnerable to ill health and premature death. Experts believe, "Those who have close personal relationships cope better with various stressors of anxiety". Social support provides a sense of belonging, security, and community. In fact, when choosing any social support network, make sure you feel comfortable with the group's beliefs, practices, and expectations. I am not saying you will never have a disagreement with your friends, family, or other social support network, remember that spending time with them should make you feel accepted, peaceful, and energized, not unhappy or anxious.

Remember support from family and friends are important to the recovery process, but it is not the cure. Getting better takes hard work, mostly from the person with the disorder, and patience from everyone involved. Like other illnesses, anxiety and related disorders can take a toll on family and friends.

So, when you learn about the disorders it will help you know what to expect from the illness and the recovery process. You should also learn when to exercise patience and when to exert a little pressure. With appropriate treatment from a mental health professional, a person can overcome an anxiety disorder which leads to a better quality of life for everyone.

"There are so many clichés associated with mental health-such as the 'fine line between lunacy and genius'-which are, on the whole, a load of rubbish."

--Jo Brand--

CLEAR YOU'RE THOUGHTS

Like most things in life letting go of negative emotions and clearing your mind is easier said than done especially for someone with mental illness. However, I hope that this will help you learn how to clear your mind in a way that works for you, and you will be able to enjoy everything life has to offer. According to Scott, Arthur of "How I Can Clear My Mind," these 4 coping skill techniques will help with anxiety and can be used for a number of mental health disorders. As we now know meditation has many uses for mental health disorders (as I have demonstrated in this book), but for now we will focus on the technique to help anxiety. Research shows that mediation can be helpful in facilitating forgiveness and letting go of negative emotions. It is very important to find a place where you can sit and relax. Then simply "observe" your surroundings. For example watch the animals as they go about their day listen or feed the birds or watch the people.

Second, mindfulness in relationship with meditation is a way of becoming fully absorbed in an activity rather than in your thoughts about other things. Study has shown, "Mindfulness is a great meditatively action for busy people." It's is said it involves slowing your mind and body down, focusing on what you need, to get relaxed to clear your mind. Try to complete one activity, such as cleaning a room, with mindfulness this can be a soothing way to clear your mind and get things you need done too. Third, writing a journaling can help you develop a topic so you can visually brainstorm solutions and examine different ways of looking at your problems which can help you to let it go. It will help you to create a time limit so you don't get stuck in your thoughts.

Forth, distract yourself to help change your focus (find a hobby). Get out and exercise with a friend. Create a project to work on that your love. Or lose yourself in a good book for a few minutes a day. This is an excellent way to bring positive active people into your life and will allow you to take a break from stress and worry.

"I was one of those people who put too much emphasis on work and career and material possessions, and it took its toll on all my relationships, on my physical health, my emotional and mental health."
--Tony Shalhoub--

STAY SOBER

According to Dooley, Arthur of "Why Alcohol Causes Anxiety," there are basically 6 reasons why alcohol consumption and hang over make many people anxious and causes anxiety to rise. I've heard a lot of people say that anxiety suffers should not drink alcohol because it makes you more nervous than you already are. However, there is a lot of evidence showing this is not simply what people are saying but it is a true fact. Alcohol may not affect all people the same, but as an anxiety sufferer, you should be aware of the consequences of alcohol consumptions. In all honesty, alcohol can affect our mood because it can affect the level of serotonin in the brain. "Serotonin is a feel good brain chemical that when in short supply can cause feeling of anxiety and depression." To add, alcohol is known to cause a drop in blood sugar that will cause dizziness, confusion, weakness, nervousness, shaking and numbness. These symptoms can most certainly trigger anxiety. Further, alcohol has been known to cause dehydration which cause nausea, dizziness, fatigue, light headedness, and muscle weakness. Experts feel these symptoms wouldn't cause anxiety but they add to a since of illness that promotes anxiety faster.

Also, researchers have documented, alcohol affects the nervous system by putting the body into a state of hyperactivity in order to counteract this effect. Hyperactivity can lead to shaking, light sound sensitivity and sleep deprivation. And, "your heart rate can become elevated as a result of consuming alcohol which can cause or palpitation false alarm and put you into a state of anxiety anticipation." Not knowing if you are having a heart attack or anxiety attack can increase your state of anxiety alone. Not only can a hard night of drinking make you lazy it can bring on headaches and create a sense of disorientation and you lose your concentration as well.

Message to the reader: If you're going to have a glass of wine with dinner I don't think you should be concerned about your anxiety. On the other hand, if you're a heavy drinker or binge drinker, then this might cause a real problem in your life and with others you love and people around you.

"A desire to be in charge of our own lives, a need for control, is born in each of us. It is essential to our mental health, and our success, that we take control."
--Robert Foster Bennett--

JOURNALING AND ANXIETY

Just like exercising journaling is another effective coping technique that can be used for most mental health illnesses. There is a lot of evidence that journaling is therapeutic especially before bedtime. People who experience anxiety tend to have very active minds, even though they aren't necessarily thinking about anything anxiety related. "It's simply a common issue that affects those with anxiety." According to Scott, Arthur of "Journaling; A Great Tool For Coping With Anxiety," when you write out your thoughts onto a permanent piece of paper, your mind takes a note of this and knows that it doesn't have to focus on it as much and eventually you'll stop thinking about it and it will stop keeping you awake. Journaling is easy to do, and is said to have a lot of benefits for reducing your anxiety level. Even if all you have is a piece of paper around you, consider using it. Here's how it's done says Scott.

First, write about your concerns and write for several minutes until you feel you have written what needs to be said. You can use anything that is comfortable for you to write on. A computer, a journal, or just a pad and paper; if you are using paper, it will be helpful if you skip a line or two for every line you use because you may want to use it later. Second, detail what is happening to you right now, describing the events that are currently causing difficulties. Keep in mind that, with anxiety, sometimes it isn't what is currently happening that is causing stress, but rather your concerns about what could happen. If this is the case for you, it's okay; you can write about what is currently happening and just note that the only part that is really stressful is the possibility of what could happen next. This in fact, may be a realization that brings some stress relief in itself. Third, write about your concerns and fears, and write in chronological order.

In other words, start with one of the stressors that is bothering now, and explore what you think will happen next, then write what you fear will happen after that.

And, write how this would affect you. Some of my clients write in their journals during group sessions, because during the group or one-on-one discussion is the only time their thought of what is bothering them occurs and when they remember what affects them we can discuss what bothers them and what coping skills is necessary to implement in their daily life right on the spot.

Note to the reader: Now that you have your thoughts in order, see what coping skills you can do to relieve some of the anxiety inside you and create your action plan today.

"When I wrote 'silver Linings,' I thought I was writing a book about the Philadelphia Eagles and male bonding, but when the book came out, it was surprising to me that the mental health community embraced it."
--Matthew Quick—

MUSIC AND ANXIETY

Music has been called 'The International Language' Even if you can't speak the language of a country, you can move, sway, dance and most of all enjoy the music of the country. Have you
No matter what kind of music you listen to, it makes your u ever heard the saying, 'Music soothes the savage beast?' It's true. There is a lot of evidence showing music can calm and revitalize us in ways even a long nap can't. And, music holds the power to raise our moods above our worries and relieve unbearable anxiety as well as perk us up if we use it with exercise or dance. With this in mind, try listening to classical music for a sense of power, soft lullaby-like music to unwind, or medium-fast music for exercise and housecleaning. When you put more music in your life it can become a powerfully enriching tool. So let's try doing something other than turning on the car radio. Here are other ways you can try. One way is to take advantage of your public library's collection of music. It's ok to have a personal favorite type of music such as rock, or jazz, but discover other music you may not think of such as country music. And if you decide you don't like that, try opera or alternative music. You won't believe how many types of music you will find once you start looking. You don't have to like all music you listen to just try to learn how to appreciate it.

In addition, you can use your IPOD or table computer so you can listen to music throughout the day or while waiting for an appointment stuck in traffic or on you lunch hour at work. It's been said by my client when they put on headphones it blocks out the stress around them and listening to the music helps them to relax. Other ways you can enjoy music is to check your local paper or look online for live music performances and go to a music concert alone or with a friend. Or, for those people who are creative you can write your own music. Expressing your emotion through music or though lyrics may be easier than having to speak how you are feeling. Remember you are writing your lyrics or music for you not for anyone else so you don't need to worry about impressing anyone.

    Also, it can be helpful to find the lyrics to one of your favorite songs and read through the lyrics and analyze why you like the song and why the words are meaningful to you. As a final point, "The bottom line is that this is a low-cost, simple and side-effect free way to use less sedative medication and reduce anxiety in mechanically-ventilated patients," said Weinert, MD., MPH., study co-author and associate professor of medicine in the University of Minnesota Medical School.

"I'm a big proponent of having a mental health component go along with whatever the physical realities are."
--Allan Thicke--

HOT SHOWER

As was previously stated, there is something about water that stops the energy of panic. Sometimes crying release it (tears). However, try taking a hot bath or shower for immediate relief of anxiety. In addition, some people drink hot soup or a hot drink (non-caffeinated) they say it can help calm them down. For many people who deal with anxiety and panic attacks in a regular basis, night time can be a difficult time of day because they are unable to fall asleep. Given these points, not getting enough sleep can take its toll on your health and well-being. It can also increase the risk of an anxiety or panic attack in the near future. Experts believe one of the most important steps you can take mentally is to simply assume that you won't sleep. This sounds like the opposite of what you are trying to accomplish, but the goal here is to break out of the pattern of assuring yourself you will fall asleep. A good night sleep isn't guaranteed, but you have to surrender your inability to sleep in order to put your mind at ease. It's been said taking a hot bath or shower allows your muscles to relax and it helps you wind down and encourage the sleep state.

Researchers at Yale University say people who take long, hot showers or baths may do so to ward off feelings of loneliness or social isolation, and say their findings could help treat mental illnesses and social phobias. "The more isolated a person feels, the more baths or showers they will take a day, the hotter they will be, and the longer they stay in the bath or shower". Interestingly, some people say holding a warm drink can make someone more trusting and generous towards others. Researchers say their findings have potential significance for the treatment of severe mental and social disorders with major public health benefits.

Just as elderly people often relocate to warmer climates, the study point out that there may be benefits to people with mental health difficulties in doing so as well.

"Most mental health professionals, including clinicians and researchers, endorse the deficit theory. They're convinced that we wage war simply because we don't know how to make love. We desperately want loving, satisfying relationships but lack the skills we need to develop them."

--David D. Burns—

BIKE RIDING

As I have said earlier in this book exercising is very beneficial for your health and mental well being. With this in mind, I am going to focus on one exercise that my client's said to be above all exercises when it comes to reducing anxiety which is biking. Research shows that biking is the perfect way to get your bloods flowing and your heart rate up. It's easier to keep up a biking routine than running or step aerobics because biking helps you tone muscle without putting strain on your joints. In addition, fitness experts believe its rhythmic motion that helps ease anxiety by focusing your attention away from stressful thoughts and providing a feeling of satisfaction after your workout session. Biking is such a diverse activity. Individuals who enjoy exercise classes can take spinning classes, and people who would rather spend time outdoors can ride their bikes on a trail or mountain biking. If you're an individual on the go, you can even save time by biking to and from work, visiting a friend or while you run errands. When searching for an exercise to reduce anxiety or any mental illness, it's important that the activity is enjoyable. When you bike, you're more likely to have fun instead of watching a timer and waiting for your workout to end. Studies have shown that the benefits of aerobic exercise increase with intensity of your exercise, so make sure you're challenging yourself when you choose your biking path. Go up steep hills and try to increase your speed. Beware of straining your back muscles as you pedal. Remember to wear protective clothes (helmet and pads) to protect your knees and elbows. You may not be able to feel the difference right away, your anxiety well decrease over time.

Also, experts believe anxiety can be relieved with a combination of lifestyle changes, such as regular exercise routine and natural remedies. Study after study has shown that working out helps reduce the negative health effects of stress. When you exercise we put our body under stress.

However, unlike the inactive stress that we feel when we are sitting at our disks, when we exercise, we actually conditions our bodies to deal with stress in the way that it was meant to deal with it. Our bodies were designed to get up and get going when life is stressful. Exercises such as biking helps relieve our body of the stress hormones and produce feel good hormones.

Studies show when you are biking riding "The repetitive action of pedaling involved in cycling can help your brain release outside stresses in the same way that mediating on a phrase or a word is used in social medical." By focusing on your pedal stoke you can block out other worries and stresses of the day, giving the brain a break from all your daily problems and have a positive outlook on tomorrow.

"Nothing happens by chance."
--Rosie O'Donnell--

DO SOMETHING FOR YOURSELF

Although most of us spend a good portion of our day taking care of family members and others, most of the time we neglect to take care of ourselves. In fact, it's been said some people feel guilty if they take the time to do something nice for themselves. For example, some of us make the choice of do they spend some time for their self or taking care of someone else's needs. It's great to know that you are taking care of other people, but it's also important to do something nice for yourself every day as well. Doing something nice for yourself doesn't have to be time-consuming or expensive. If we think about it, some of the nicest moments of your life don't have any kind of cost associated with them at all. The important thing is to choose something each day that will make you feel happy and well help you take care of yourself. In ether event, don't ever feel bad that you're allowing yourself to enjoy some free time and dedicating it to your happiness. Remember you deserve to take some time off and should feel ok about it. People who do not stop and take a moment for themselves can become depressed or frustrated with their lives which can produce anxiety towards the people around them.

Also, it's been said trying to maintain good health can be hard and expensive to do, but if you remain positive and reward yourself now and then, it's beneficial for your mental state. However, because we are different individuals you will find everyone has different ideas as to what makes them happy, your list of good deeds for yourself would probably not be the same as what your friend, partner, or child would choose for themselves. But since you know yourself better than anybody else you would be more qualified to choose something that will make you happy. This is why for some people an expensive present purchased for you by someone else sometimes isn't as satisfying as the small treat you buy or do for yourself.

For example, your daily "take care of "yourself" moment might include doing something healthy for yourself such as taking a long walk, biking or being around good people. Or it could be something that would bring you long lasting happiness such as adding your favored scented throughout your home so that you can enjoy it every time you walk through your house. And, if you want to take yourself to lunch at a favorite restaurant now and then, you should do it.

Or, treat yourself to a new bottle of perfume, go to a football game, buy a new suit, or for you gardeners try an afternoon gardening in the yard. The possibilities are endless. After all, it's usually the little things in life that makes us happy.

> *"Mental health is seen as a massive drag to have to write about-worthy, dull. Something you should 'have' to read/write about."*
>
> --Caitlin Moran--

GET MOTIVATED AND THINK POSITIVE

Research shows, if you're suffering from anxiety or any other mental health issues, motivation is something you'll find hard to achieve. According to Dich, Arthur of "All Things Depression: Strategies For Anxiety, Depression, Stress, And Anger," states, "If your anxiety is at full swing, you probably find yourself so mentally exhausted from all the thinking that you're left with nothing in the tank to do anything else." Whatever is causing your anxiety it can take all your energy and strength out of your body. If you can find a way to gather together the strength to go talk to a therapist, you'll probably find that any homework they give you turns into a chore. You then can end up feeling like a failure and start to engage in negative self-talk and behavior and the cycle downward continues. Experts believe, when lack of motivation is combined with mental health issues, a person may resign themselves to accept their state rather than allowing positive interventions to create a better, healthy frame of mind.

To add, it's been said thinking positive is just the beginning to a wonderful life and once you begin to learn how to think positive the universe will start to change for you and opportunities will become more available. Believe it or not, your finances will increase because you're thinking actually become clearer, you will hear the answer to your problem and you can make better decisions. Also, along with a positive life, you will attract other positive people in your life that will have the integrity, honesty and will be decent to you and other. These are the positive aspect we're talking about. There is a lot of evidence showing when we think positive, things will be better and your life will just be a whole lot easier.

Here are other benefits that come along with thinking positive. Not only will you become a happier person, you won't be so depressed and by thinking positive you can decrease your anxiety and control it. If you want a happier and joyful life, think positive and get motivated. Here's how to start on a happier and joyful life.

First, develop a successful attitude. Get motivated and know yourself. "To truly understand what we are made of we must test ourselves and learn our personal strengths and weaknesses and discover what you are good at in life and apply this self-knowledge to live your life based on your strengths. Find ways to improve yourself that will help you overcome your weaknesses. Get motivated now and go into action. Do what ever it takes to improve your life (legally, morally and ethically of course). "One way to get motivated is to read uplifting articles or books from successful people." I can't stress enough how important it is to feed your mind, body and spirit with good news, success stories and encouraging talks.

"There are lots of people with mental health disabilities, and that's just the way their life is; it's not like you see it in the movies."

--Andy Behman--

HIGHER POWER

As was previously stated, most people will seek prayer when their anxiety strikes or for comfort and others who don't pray will seek their higher power through chanting or meditation. It's been said this process allows them to feel the spirit of their higher power flow through their body to help rejuvenate the soul. According to research the meaning of "higher power" is unclear. It means something different to each of us. According to Almeida, Arthur of What is Higher Power? Suggest, some people accredit the existence of a personal higher power to their guardian angel, guides, ascended masters (such as Jesus, Buddha, and Moses), and even various gods. "Some like to call it their subconscious. Almeida treats the possibility of a higher power as a mystical and metaphysical matter. Sometimes he likes to refer to the higher power as a "great power". This phrase communicates the immenseness of this mysterious god-like being. "Perhaps this being could be seen as both a higher and greater power."

In other words, part of the reason why my clients reach out for their higher power because it's been said a greater power is an enteric being or entity which looks out for the well-being an individual. Most people believe that each of us has a higher or greater power watching over us. There are many descriptions for this entity we call the greater power. In Almeida own exploration into mysticism and metaphysics he discovered what he believe to be the true nature of the entity we call the greater power or higher power. First, the greater power is an intelligent entity. It is a vibrational energy like all entitles that resides in the infinite multi-verse. Thorough divine illumination, he believes that the Great War is a collective being composed of each human's past lives. This makes the greater power a personal companion of sorts.

Each of our past lives belongs to us and we belong to them. "We are united in power with our ancestors". Our ancestors will always be with use to help use through any situation and to comfort us.

"I try to make my bed every day for mental health. Coming home to an unmade bed or room with clothes all over will depress me."

--David Alan Grier--

RELAXATION

For many of us, relaxation means sitting in front of the TV watching your favorite TV show at the end of a stressful day. But this does little to reduce the damaging effects of anxiety. To effectively fight anxiety, we need to activate the body's natural relaxation response. You can do this by practicing relaxation techniques such as deep breathing, meditation, rhythmic exercise, and yoga says Robinson and Smith, Arthur of Relaxation Techniques for Stress Relief. Fitting one or more of these activities into your life can help reduce everyday stress or anxiety and boost your energy and mood. Anxiety is necessary for life. You need a certain amount of anxiety for creativity, learning, and your very survival. Anxiety is only harmful when it become overwhelming and interrupts the healthy state of equilibrium that your nervous system needs to remain in balance. Unfortunately, overwhelming anxiety has become an increasingly common characteristic of contemporary life. Some people say they work better under stress and anxiety. Experts believe, "When anxiety throws your nervous system out of balance, relaxation techniques can bring it back into a balanced state by producing the relaxation response, a state of deep calmness." Relaxation techniques are an important component for anxiety disorders and other mental health disorders.

In addition, for example, if you have a fear of public speaking, part of your treatment may involve the practice of deep breathing and muscle relaxation while imaging giving a speech. Research shows Diaphragmatic Breathing or deep breathing is the practice of expanding your diaphragm as you breathe, so that your stomach rises and fall instead of your chest. During an anxiety attack, you are more likely to take shallow breathes, which contributes to symptoms of anxiety says Robinson and Smith.

There is no single relaxation technique that will work for everyone. It's been suggested, when choosing a relaxation technique consider your specific needs, preferences, fitness level, and the way you tend to react to anxiety. The right relaxation technique is the one that resonates with you, fits your lifestyle, and is able to focus your mind and break up your everyday thoughts in order to bring out the relaxation response.

> *"I'm convinced that we can shape a different future for this country as it relates to mental health and as it relates to suicide."*
>
> *--David Satcher--*

Chapter 2

MANAGING DEPRESSION

More and more people are feeling a wide range of symptoms of depression. There is evidence showing everyone experiences the normal ups and downs of life, and everyone feels sad or has "the blues" sometimes. But if helplessness and hopelessness won't go away, you may have depression. Depression makes it rough for you to function and feel "normal" like you once did. Just getting through the day can be a lot of work. It's been said that depression can confine you to your home, and not wanting to have visitors. This can lead to other mental health symptoms if not treated says Sega Arthur of Depression. However, no matter how hopeless you feel, it is some things you can do to help you get better. It is important to know the signs and symptoms of depression so you will know when you need to seek help and this chapter will help you to be aware of them. According to the Diagnostic and Statistical Manual of Mental Disorders, some of the signs and symptoms of depression include but not limited is the feeling of helplessness and hopelessness, having a negative outlook on life, the loss of interest in daily activities with no interest in former hobbies, social activities, or sex. Also, other symptoms are losing the ability to feel joy and pleasure, appetite and weight change, significant weight loss or weight gain, a change of more than 5 percent of body weight in a month. And, some people can experience a sleep change and have symptoms of insomnia. This can result to walking in the early hours of the morning, or oversleeping, feeling anger or irritability, feeling agitated, restless, or even violent.

In addition, the facts show you can develop a low tolerance level by developing a short temper, and everything and everyone starts to get on your nerves, lost of energy, feeling fatigued, sluggish, and physical drained, your whole body may feel heavy, and even small tasks are exhausting or take longer to complete or self-loathing, strong feelings of worthlessness or guilt. Research discovered other systems are reckless behavior, you engage in bad behavior such as substance abuse, compulsive gambling, reckless driving, or dangerous sports.

Lastly, you have concentration problems, trouble focusing, making decisions, or remembering things, unexplained arches and pains, an increase in physical complaints. If you recognize the signs of depression in yourself or a loved one, take some time to discover the many treatment options in the chapter. There is evidence showing when you're depressed, it can feel like you'll never get out from under a dark cloud. However, even the most severe depression is treatable. So, if your depression is keeping you from living the life you want to, don't hesitate to seek help. Learning about your depression treatment options will help you decide what approach is right for you. From therapy to holistic approach, medication to healthy lifestyle changes, there are many effective treatments that can help you overcome depression and reclaim your life found in this book.

TALK ABOUT IT

It is very important to have a discussion with a family member that you know will be supportive regarding your depression, says Richard C. Shelton, MD, department of psychiatry, Vanderbilt University School of Medicine in Nashville, Tenn., studies has shown, there are a number of reasons why talking about depression with your loved ones is both necessary and helpful. For people who have never experienced depression, it can be hard to understand your symptoms. Dr. Shelton says, explaining your condition and depression symptoms can help them understand the reasons why you've been feeling and acting the way you have which will enable them to explain them to you, and they'll be more able to recognize your depressive episodes when you can't and let you know when you are unaware of what you are doing. Sometimes it is hard to see something you are experiencing when you are in the moment. Your family member will be able to support you through your symptoms. Being open about depression symptoms can also help remove some of the stigma attached to mental illness, such as calling it a weakness. Dr. Shelton suggests you encourage family members or other people you know to do the same if they become depressed.

On the other hand, Shelton warns, "sharing with family members is not with some risk, some people may not be all that welcoming of the idea. It may be that they don't understand that depression is a medical condition and can't be controlled without treatment or they just refuse to admit that depression is a part of their family. Most of my clients stated their families refuse to admit that depression is a part of their family because they can't face the stigmas behind mental health. At worst, some family members may say that it is just laziness or a lack of faith says Shelton. It is suggested that you exercise some judgment when deciding whom to share information about your depression.

If it's a family member or friend ask yourself if that person will offer the support that you need. Most of the time a treatment plan for major depression often involves a combination of medication, lifestyle changes, and taking therapy, such as cognitive therapy and interpersonal therapy, so you can better understand what is causing your depression.

Also, this is a good time to take some holistic measures. Taking cognitive therapy and interpersonal therapy involve working with a therapist to develop the coping skill that will create healthier, more proactive thoughts.

"Self-esteem is as important to our well-being as legs are to a table. It is essential for physical and mental health and for happiness."

--Louise Hart--

SEEK UNDERSTANDING

Knowing what causes your depression can help you to be aware of the people you share your space with and your environment around you. This can help you avoid the things that will bring you to a down state of mind. There are combinations of factors that may contribute to depression. According to the National Institute of Mental Health, people with a family history of depression may be more likely to develop depression than those whose families do not have the illness. People with depression have different brain chemistry than those without the illness says NIMH. This can allow stress, loss of a love one, a difficult relationship, or any stressful situation to trigger depression. Depression does not affect all people in the same way. Depression affects different people in different ways. For example, research shows women experience depression more often than men because of their biological, life cycle, and hormonal factors that are unique to women may be linked to women's higher depression rate. Women with depression typically have symptoms of sadness, worthlessness, and guilt. On the other hand, men with depression are more likely to be very tired, irritable, and sometimes even angry. They may lose interest in work or activities they once enjoyed, and have sleep problems. And, older adults with depression may have less obvious symptoms, or they may be less likely to admit to feelings of sadness or grief. They also are more likely to have medical conditions like heart disease or stroke, which may cause or contribute to depression, says NIMH

In addition, there is evidence showing certain medications also can have side effects that contribute to depression. Further, children with depression may pretend to be sick, refuse to go to school, cling to a parent, or worry that a parent may die.

Older children or teens may get into trouble at school and be irritable. Because these signs can also be part of normal mood swings associated with certain childhood stages, it may be difficult to accurately diagnose a young person with depression. Everyone occasionally feels blue or sad. But these feelings are usually short-lived and pass within a couple of days.

Also, when you have depression, it interferes with daily life and cause pain for both you and those who care about you. Depression is a common but serious illness. Many people with depressive illness never seek treatment. But the majority (even those with the most severe depression) can get better with treatment. Medications, psychotherapies, holistic approach, and other coping methods can effectively treat people with depression says NIMH

"Studies have shown that inmate participation in education, vocational and job training, prison work skills development, drug abuse, mental health and other treatment programs, all reduce recidivism, significantly."
--Bobby Scott--

LIST SOLUTIONS

Some individuals feel thinking and listing solutions for their depression helps them to stay focus and concentrate on how to feel better. It's been suggested to try to list every way that you can think to overcome your depression. Don't worry about how unrealistic an idea may seem. Write down anything and everything. It may take some time but it will be worth it. The best solutions to your depression are likely to be the ones you think of yourself. This is because nobody really knows your situations as well as you do. It may help if you consider how you solved similar problems in the past; what your friends or family would suggest or how you would like to see yourself tackling the problem. After you choose a solution, next you need to take the best solution from your list and think carefully about each option. It is useful to go through all the reasons "for" and "against" each idea. It can be easier if you created two columns. This will help you to make a good decision and select the best solution. After this if you are still unsure, maybe a couple of approaches seem equally good. Try to pick one to begin with and if it doesn't work then you can always go back and try out a different one later.

Also, It's been suggested to break down your solution, it will help you carry out your chosen solutions; it is useful to break it down into small steps because this can make it easier and more manageable to follow through. The number of steps required will vary depending on the solution and how complex it is. For example; someone in debt may have decided to try and resolve their problem by getting a part time job. This would require several steps. First, you will have to buy a newspaper with job adverts; second, choose which jobs to apply for; third, create a resume sending it out; fourth, buy interview clothes and preparing answers for potential interview questions.

To follow the steps required to carry out your solution just take them one at a time and go at your own pace and don't allow yourself to feel rushed. If you start to feel rushed just stop and take a few hours to step back from working on your solution and come back when you are ready.

Once you have completed all the steps. You should review the outcome, and once you have successfully resolved your problem then great. If the problem still exists don't give up keep trying other solutions that is described in this book to help you with your depression.

"Big brother is on the march. A plan to subject all children to mental health screening is underway, and the pharmaceuticals are gearing up for bigger sales of psychotropic drugs."
--Phyllis Schlafly--

HOTLINE

There is a lot of evidence that indicates calling a hotline for depression can save your life. Even hotlines that are listed as suicide hotline welcome calls from individuals who are depressed. The fact is if you call a hotline you will not get turn away if you are someone who is not suicidal. The people on the other end of the phone understands the importance of preventing someone from becoming suicidal that's why they will talk to someone who has not yet reach that place in their mind. A person should call a hotline if they need reassurance that he or she is not alone in their problems and to get comfort that other people understand and care about your problems.

In addition, sometimes you can be afraid to talk to someone you know because you are afraid they will be judgmental. When calling a hotline you don't have to worry about that because the person on the other end is a non judgmental person if you need to talk to someone outside of your family and friends calling a hotline is a great outlet. The hotline worker will provide a kind, listening ear and understanding of what you are going through and this alone sometimes lower your level of depression and allow you to get the rest you need. Most hotlines operate 24/7 and most are free. For most of these hotlines, there is never a bad time to call. The National Suicide Prevention Lifeline number is (1-800-273-TALK). The important thing for anyone who suffers from depression to know is help is available. Someone who understands what you are going through is just a call away or available via e-therapy @, http://therapist2013.wix.com/e-therapy, internet chats, or email. If you are battling depression please reach out for help for your sake and the sake of those who love you.

One of the main reasons that depression can turn deadly is the loneliness and despair that many of its victims feel. Those suffering from depression may feel a sense of isolation, a sense that nobody understands or cares to understand what they are going through. Just one call to a hotline can help depression victims achieve immediate personal contact with someone who has been trained to assist the suicidal and the lonely. The thing to remember is there is always someone to talk to just a phone call away.

"A library is a place that is a repository of information and gives every citizen equal access to it. That includes health information and mental health information. It's a community space. It's a place of safety, a haven from the world."
--Neil Gaiman--

TELEVISION

There is a lot of evidence that shows television is a way for people with depression to disconnect from the effects of depression for a while. Sometimes active watching in moderation is helpful. At other times, passive watching can become a form of self medication. Either way, those with depression should monitor how long and what they watch on television. It's been suggested to watch a good comedy when feeling down. It is always good to laugh and it can be contagious. Laughing also is referred to as and exercises for you inter organs. When you laugh it shakes you all over in and out of your body. The best time to watch television is when you are feeling stable or "up" not "down". Television tends to trigger or deepen depression if it is watched for long hours at one sitting. It can become a passive exercise of occasionally turning into disconnected images and sounds. Then the sensation from the television acts like a depressant. According to Psychiatric Times, "adolescents exposed to television had significantly greater odds of developing depression for each hour of daily exposure." People who fight depression sometimes self medicate themselves by watching television as a soothing distraction.

In addition, it's been suggested that you determine how long to watch television in advance by setting an alarm on your phone or oven timer to remind you your time is up. Half an hour to two hours is a reasonable time to watch television in one sitting without experiencing a negative effect says Psychiatric Times. Researchers discovered it is helpful to choose your shows wisely. Such as watching sitcoms, light dramas, action, educational, sports, arts, or music talent shows. On the other hand, dark sad or violent shows can trigger a mood swing.

Also, know what kind of shows is better to watch at night before going to bed and in the afternoon watch television that's engaging. For example, game shows, such as "Family Feud," "Jeopardy," "The price is right" and "wheel of Fortune," experience it all; winning, losing, anticipation, excitement, disappointment, enthusiasm and inspiration. This will help prevents passive television watching. Since game shows are regularly scheduled, they can become part of a routine and only last for half an hour. Any show that stimulates healthy emotions is usually a good indication that it's a depression safe show.

"I don't believe you have to have eating disorders and mental illness to screw up."
--Kirstie Alley--

http://therapist2013.wix.com/e-therapy

READ

A lot of my clients stated reading helps with their depression and here is why. Studies have shown, reading is used as a form of depression therapy. Most people have never heard of bibliotherapy. Reading books for medical treatment was proved effective for wounded veterans in World War II says Folk-Williams, Arthur of Reading as A Form of Depression Therapy. Moreover, Bibliotherapy (another name for reading) also seems to be helpful for depression says John Folk-Williams. Bibliotherapy or reading therapy is a therapy used for an individual suffering from depression. It is recommended to reads self-help books (such as the one you are reading now) and other motivational books in between therapies to speed up your recovery. Controlled clinical trials have shown that bibiliotherapy can give results comparable to that of drug therapy or psychotherapy. And, patients in bibliotherapy recovered faster from depression than those on conventional therapy, says Follk-Williams. After bibliotherapy it is said most people had a better outlook on life. Bibliotherapy is also useful as a complementary coping skill to speed up the recovery along with conventional therapy.

According to John Folk-Williams, Bibliotherapy can be administered in one of two ways.

1. The therapists can prescribe a self-help book for their patients to read between therapy sessions to increase the speed of learning and recovery (Complementary therapy)

1. Individuals suffering from depression or anxiety can be given a self-help book to read as a self-administered treatment without any other drug therapy or psychotherapy. (stand-alone therapy)

To add, the big problem with the drug therapy and other conventional therapies for depression is the dropout rate. Patients quit taking medication because of the side effects and stop going to therapy because there depression slowly shows back up. According to Folk-Williams, the percentage of patients who dropped out of the bibliotherapy studies was very small (10 percent) compared to the published outcome studies using drugs or psychotherapy which typically have dropout rates from 15 to over 54 percent. The patients developed significantly more positive attitudes and thinking patterns after bibliotherapy. It is said the bibliotherapy helped the patients to defeat depression by changing the negative thinking patterns that caused it.

"Mental Illness is nothing to be ashamed of, but stigma and bias shame us all."

--Bill Clinton--

MUSIC AND DEPRESSION

As we previously stated, music has the power to influence people's emotions; it can make you happy, sad, or angry. So let's look in detail at how it helps with depression. Research shows music can also aid in the recovery of mental illnesses. The Geriatric Mental Health Department of the Chhatarati Shahuju Maharaj Medical University in India is starting a music therapy clinic to treat elderly patients with mental disorders (like dementia) nearly 5% of elderly people older than 60 suffer from dementia. Not only can music therapy help people with mental illnesses, but playing an instrument and being a part of an ensemble can help too. The Concert Ensembles is a group of 50 musicians from Cambridge, Massachusetts, who are all living with a mental illness. The group helps musicians move away from the mental patient role into a new identity as a professional musician and performer. Moreover, a recent review of research by Cochrane researchers indicates that music therapy can help with depression. Millions of people suffer from depression with the only treatments being psychotherapy, medications and some herbal substances. The researchers looked at five studies. Four of these indicated a decrease in symptoms of depression while the fifth did not. The researchers concluded that there was enough evidence to warrant further study on how music effect depression. Music is a powerful thing, it consists of sound waves that contain information that is processed by our nervous systems and this information in turn affects our minds and bodies. Music has the power to draw out emotions and "move" people. It has been said it may also have the power to heal.

Also, researchers have documented how music therapy is used to cure depression. Music is not only a way to recreate ourselves, but it is extremely beneficial for our mental health. Music therapy is used to heal depression.

When we listen to music of our choice daily our immune system is strengthened a lot. The human body does not produce the hormones which cause depression if we listen to the music daily. Some people also meditate with the help of music. For example, sit at a calm place and wear a good quality headphone. Then play music of your choice in slow volume and close your eyes. Now realize how much soothing this mixture of music therapy and meditation can be. You will feel strong and happy from within. You can listen to the music of your choice anytime anywhere. You will feel a kind of satisfaction after listening to the music. You will also feel that your life is full of happiness.

So I hope you will now listen to the music of your choice daily as a coping skill to get rid of depression and for your mental well being.

"Normal is an illusion. What is normal for the spider is chaos for the fly."

--Morticia Addams--

JOURNALING AND DEPRESSION

I talked about how journaling can reduce anxiety and most mental illnesses. Here are some examples of how journaling your own success story helps to relive depression. First, you should understand that being depressed is certainly no way to dealing with hardships. Research shows being depressed have mental as well as physical repercussions. Facts shows depression always adds to your anxiety levels and never lets you stay at peace or stay cool, calm and composed. Also, you can never live a "normal" life and enjoy it to the maximum. However, being depressed is no way of finding a solution to your problems, it only waste your time and energies which can be spent in doing something constructive or maybe finding a possible solution to your problem. It's been said the rule of life is to get going when the going gets tough. So try journaling your own success story. You write the script to your life and make it as happy and positive as you would like it to be. You might remember a shift in mood but you won't remember your depression. What you write about will manifest itself into you life. So write it down and read it everyday

To add, I talk about journaling a lot because it is a powerful tool and plays an active role in your recovery for depression and any other mental health illness. Journaling is an excellent way of recovering from depression. The facts show there are two key objectives to keep in mind while you are journaling; one, recapturing the moment, because thoughts and activities can fly by quickly. Two, reflect on the moment, spend a few minutes of a day writing a journal is an opportunity to slow down, and look back and revisit the events of the day, describing not only what happened, but what you remember thinking or feeling. This can provide you useful insight into how you see yourself and the world around you. This knowledge can help you put together a treatment plan for yourself as well.

Also, it's been said journaling is a great self-teaching tool because it provides a safe environment for not only looking at what happened during the day, but examining how changing your thoughts or behaviors might have brought about a different outcome (hindsight). Many people find that once they've recounted the day's events, they can also spend a few minutes journaling about the lessons of the day, and practicing alternative ways to react to stress, handle relationships and recognize and appreciate life's positive moments. It's been said by University of Michigan Depression Center, that journaling can have a positive impact on both physical and mental health, and can make psychotherapy more effective.

"Mental illness is so much more complicated than any pill that any mortal could invent."
--Elizabeth Wurtzel--

GRATITUDE LIST

When depression hits us, it's difficult to think of anything we should be grateful for. According to the Law of Attraction having a gratitude list will shift your thinking and create positive energy in your life. It's been said being grateful can improve your outlooks on life, create a better atmosphere in and out of your home, improve relationships with others and ourselves, decrease negative feelings, help us cope with stress, and improve the quality of our overall lives. The facts show finding a few things you are grateful for in a day is simple, but the challenge is to keep listing things that you are grateful for. Researchers say that it takes 40 days to change how some parts of your brain works. So, after 40 days of working at being grateful, your brain is newly rewired to think thoughts of gratefulness more easily. This process can apply to any habit or addiction. One of the best ways to create a gratitude list is to start by writing three or more things you are grateful for everyday. It gets interesting as the days go by. For example, start by writing, "I'm thankful for…"at the top of the paper, and then write the dates and/or days of the week (you can make it quick by just writing M for Monday and, T for Tuesday, etc) for the next 40 days, leaving space to write a few things you are grateful for every day.

All in all, this is very similar to journaling but you focus more on what you are grateful for. Having all the dates/days already written on paper may encourage you to write something down each day or it's been said creating a gratitude board can be equally helpful. This can be a chalkboard or a white eraser board you have on your fridge etc. Writing down what you are thankful for on board will help you remember what you are grateful for throughout the day. If you're looking to improve your family life, try having your family write what they are grateful for before dinner.

Most families list what they are grateful for or speak publicly around the dinner table on Thanksgiving so lets try to incorporate it into are everyday life. Just make a commitment to say to yourself what you are grateful for each day. It is very easy to forget to do it. If you try this and forget a day, hang a sign up for yourself in spots you are sure to see every day that says "I'm grateful for… It might be challenging on your darkest day but I'm sure you can find something to be grateful for. It can be for something as simple as reading this book because it means you at least have the strength to try and improve your life, which you can and will as long as you keep hope alive.

"Be thankful for what you have; you'll end up having more. If you concentrate on what you don't have, you will never, ever have enough."
--Oprah Winfrey--

CRAFTS

As I have said, finding or developing hobbies is a helpful coping skill for mental illness. One hobby that was mention over and over in my group is crafts. It is a proven fact, that moderately busy people are happy people. Having something to do in your spare time can really help prevent depression. Studies have shown making crafts or showing others how to do crafts can help a depressed person. Experts believe scrap booking is an excellent way to help with depression. For example, make a scrapbook of happy and cheerful things in your life. Also, colors can help boost our moods in all areas of our lives. It is said to use bright colors like yellow which brings about positivity and happiness, light blue which allows energy to be peaceful and relaxed, and green welcomes in harmony and stability. Some people wear their favorite color, paint a room an energy boosting color or even drive your favorite color car. Red is said to open the door for passion energies and enhances metabolism, orange is an energy boost and self confidence, white represents purity with an ease of energies.

In addition, modern science tells us one of the best cures for depression is good old-fashioned work with your hands. Pottery has kept most people clicking along, even during the Midwestern winters, which is said to normally make you feel dull and down. And, research suggests that when we immerse ourselves in activities involving planning, anticipation, and self-forgetting movement, such as gardening, crafting, or even working on a car engine, we not only come back into the moment but also reduce stress and combat depression. Also, hands-on work is said to satisfy our primal craving to create solid objects; it could also be an cure to our cultural depression, says neuroscientist Kelly Lambert, chair of the psychology department at Virginia's Randolph-Macon College and author of "Lifting Depression."

Lambert had a moment while reading "Little House on the Prairie" to her daughter. She was thinking of the contrast between her own push-button lifestyle and Ma Ingalls's day-in, day-out labor, she realized that hard physical working producing tangible results might be a source of pleasure. Ma's chores were collecting rainwater for baths, sewing every article of clothing for her husband and children were no laughing matter. And yet, Lambert came to think, those tasks were for the survival of Ma and Family, they were also probably quite rewarding for her mental health. What is your favorite craft?

"It's ok to talk about mental illness. No one should be embarrassed about it."

--Nicla Campbell--

CHALLENGE NEGATIVE THINKING

When negative thoughts hit your brain, it's tempting to struggle with them and try to shove a more positive thought in your head. In the day-to-day reality this doesn't really work. Your emotions can have a tough grip on your negative thoughts, so the best thing to do is to imagine yourself emotionally "Letting go" of them before depression accurse. Research shows the letting go approach is used in yoga and meditation to help a person stay focused on the present. When thinking about getting rid of your negativity, you might start by trying to push those thoughts out of your mind, stop and consider a different approach, something that would go along with meditation and yoga. Fighting against something usually takes a lot more energy than avoiding a fight in the first place. Instead of pushing your negative thoughts out, you can acknowledge and release them. And when they come back, acknowledge that they are still coming and release them again. Look in the mirror and tell them what they need to do. You don't try to wrestle them out of your mind; you just let them go on their way. Also, depression puts a negative spin on everything, including the way you see yourself, your situations, and your expectations for the future. You have to do more than just think positive happy thoughts, and wishful thinking won't cut it all the time. Remember, everything needs a replacement. So, the trick is to replace negative thoughts with more balance thoughts. Think outside of the box and ask yourself would you say what you're thinking about yourself to someone else. If not, stop being so hard on yourself. Think about less harsh statements that offer more realistic descriptions. Allow yourself to be less than perfect.

In addition, research shows, many depressed people are perfectionists, holding themselves to impossibly high standards and then beating themselves up when they fail to meet them.

To battle this source of self-imposed stress you will have to challenge your negative ways of thinking. Also, I can't stress this enough to socialize and surround yourself with positive people as much as you can. Find out how people who always look on the bright side deal with challenges, even minor ones, for example not being able to find a parking space. Then consider how you would react in the same situations. Even if you have to pretend, try to adopt their optimism and persistence in the face of difficulty. Be aware of what triggers your negative thoughts when you're in a good mood then try to avoid them. Consider if the negativity was really necessary, then ask yourself if there's another way to look at the situation. For example, let's say your friend was short with you and you automatically assumed that it was something you done. Look at all the possibilities. It could be possible they are just having a bad day.

"I'll never forget how the depression and loneliness felt good and bad at the same time. Still does."
--Henry Rollins--

TAKE A BREAK

Study has shown taking a break from your everyday life is a way of treating depression. But for most people it is hard to take a break from their busy schedule. For example, you have a crappy job or no job, hated your education or wasn't doing anything, didn't have a good love life/social life and was getting so down about life, and decided to one day leave your normal life to go traveling somewhere for a certain amount of time? Another example, Dave Chappell walked off his job and went to Africa for awhile because of the pressure around him. It probably wouldn't help people who have severe chemical depression very much. However, there are some people who get depressed from triggers created by bad circumstances. Some people say it get better after they have taken a good break which allowed them to have a breather and think about things, and be in a different and more positive environment and around more positive people. Just remember depression can be very devastating and sometimes you just need a break from your life to decompress. Many people say solo traveling have a huge effect on boosting self esteem and confidence. It is recommended if you get the chance.

With that said, being on your own in a strange place might be very lonely if you're not used to it and feeling a bit depressed for chemical reasons. It is recommended that you take a short trip-nothing fancy-just a week somewhere inexpensive. If you feel less stressed and depressed during this time, then yes it's situational and by all means start saving your money and take yourself to wonderland before you're too old. In addition, you can't force yourself to have fun or experience pleasure just by choosing to do things that you used to enjoy. For example, you can pick up a former hobby or a sport you used to like as well as express yourself creatively through music, art or writing; or go out with a friend; or take a day trip to a museum.

Depression can make you feel like you don't want to do anything so you will have to push yourself to do things, even when you don't feel like it. You might be surprised at how much better you feel once you're out in the world. Even if your depression doesn't lift immediately, you'll gradually feel more upbeat and energetic as you make time for fun activities and eventually your depression will disappear.

"Mental illness leaves a huge legacy, not just for the person suffering it but for those around them."

--Lysette Anthony--

EXERCISE AND DEPRESSION

As has been noted, how exercising helps your mental health, here is how exercise helps with depression. Many studies show, people who exercise regularly benefit with a positive boost in mood and lower rates of depression. One of the most important psychological benefits of exercise when you have depression is improved self-esteem with regular physical activity. Research shows, when you exercise, your body release chemicals called endorphins. These endorphins interact with the receptors in your brain that reduce your perception of pain. It is said endorphins also trigger a positive feeling in the body, similar to that of morphine. For example, the feeling that follows a run or workout is often described as "euphoric". That feeling, know as a "runner's high." It also can be accompanied by a positive outlook on life. Experts believe endorphins act as analgesics; they reduce the perception of pain because they also act as sedatives. There is a lot of evidence showing endorphins are manufactured in your brain, spinal cord, and many other parts of your body and are released in response to brain chemical called neurotransmitters. Experts believe the neuron receptors endorphins found in use are the same ones that are found in some pain medicines. However, unlike with morphine, the activation of these receptors by the body's endorphins does not lead to addiction or depression and has no side effects. Regular exercise has been proven to ward off feelings of depression.

In addition, research has shown that exercise is an effective but often underused treatment for mild to moderate depression. It appears that any form of exercise can help depression because a strong social support is important for those with depression, that's why joining a group exercising class may be beneficial.

In doing so, you will benefit from the physical activity and emotional comfort as well as knowing that others are supportive of you. For most people, it is ok to start an exercise program without checking with a health care provider. However, if you have not exercised in a while, and over the age of 50, or have a medical condition, contact your health care provider before starting any exercise program.

Fitness experts believe exercise also has these added health benefits: It strengthens your heart, it increases energy levels, it lowers blood pressure, it improves muscle tone and strength, it strengthens and builds bones, it helps reduce body fat, and it makes you look fit and healthy. It is suggested before you begin an exercise program for depression, here are some question you should consider: what physical activities do you enjoy? Do you prefer group or individual activities? What program best fit your schedule? Do you have physical conditions that limit your choice of exercise? What goals do you have in mind? Once these questions are answer you are ready to choose your exercise routine. Have a good work out.

"Normal is nothing more than a cycle on a washing machine."
--Whoopi Goldberg--

HEALTHY SELF-ESTEEM

To build a healthy self-esteem the most important thing is that you do something positive and constructive. You might start by getting yourself some paper and a pen and make headings for all the factors previously described: environmental, interpersonal, physical/medical, etc. Then, make a list of any problems, concerns or negative feelings you have that relate to each of the areas. It also helps to identify which of the areas are sources of strength, support, and give you positive feelings. Depression can leave you feeling helpless and out of control of your life, your thoughts, feelings, and behaviors. The goal is to get to the point where you feel like you can do something to improve your situation and life to help build your self-esteem. So any changes you can make for the better, even if they may not "fix" the depression or make it go away immediately, are definitely worth doing. Go over each area and do your own self-assessment, and then write down what you think it would take to help the situation. Most people's thoughts and feelings about themselves fluctuate somewhat based on their daily experiences. Such as, the grade you get on an exam, how your friends treat you, or ups and downs in a romantic relationship can all have a temporary impact on how you feel about yourself.

To add, it's been said your self-esteem is something more fundamental than the normal ups and downs associated with situational changes. For people with good self-esteem, normal ups and downs may lead to temporary fluctuations in how they feel about themselves, but only to a limited extent. In contrast, for people with poor self-esteem (that can sometimes come with mental illness), these ups and downs drastically impact the way they see themselves. People with poor self-esteem often rely on how they are doing in the present to determine how they feel about themselves.

They need positive external experiences to counteract the negative feelings and thoughts that constantly plague them. Even then, the good feeling is usually temporary. Healthy self-esteem is based on our ability to assess ourselves accurately and still be accepting of who we are. In other words, this means being able to acknowledge our strengths and weaknesses and at the same time recognize that we are worthy and worthwhile says The University of Texas, Healthy Self-Esteem.

"I want to show that the dividing lines between sanity and mental illness have been drawn in the wrong place."
--Anthony Storr--

DON'T WORRY BE HAPPY

When you are depressed, happiness seems impossible but you couldn't be more wrong. Experts believe, as long as your depression is not due to a chemical imbalance (which is often not the case) these 6 steps will help you feel happier by breaking your negative thoughts and the hold it has over you says Perera, Arthur of Cure for Depression.

1. Gratitude: think of your life right now. What good things are there to be thankful for? Start listing them on a piece of paper or just go over them in your head. The fact that you can find many positive things in your life no matter how depressed you may feel is comforting and will change your mood (For more information on Gratitude, go to the Gratitude List in this chapter).
2. Pause in the moment: if you stop for one moment and forget the future and the past and concentrate on now and live in the moment, look around and ask yourself what is everything like now, you will see that there are no problems or worries in the present.
3. Instead of you always thinking negatively start to expect something positive. Change can be good. (For more information go to Get motivated and Think Positive in chapter 1).
4. No matter how bad things appear you can always find something positive. Try a positive doing at the end of your sentences when you hear yourself begin to complain.
5. Stop saying "I can't" realize that there are few things you can't do mostly what you are saying is that you don't want to do something. Examine why this is so; maybe it's just fear.
6. Start imagining things improving in your life. What you can see as possible, is possible. If you dream something

you can make it real. The only thing stopping you is your thinking and your fear.

Also, it has been shown that of all the things that man is looking for the most important is happiness. I believe when the Unite Sates Declaration of Independence was written, "Life Liberty and the Pursuit of Happiness," someone knew that happiness was going to be something that we all desperately need to find and maintain for a healthier life. If you think about this you'll see that everything you want is related to your happiness. What I mean is that whatever you think you want …it really boils down to what you think will make you happy.

Many people believe that happiness comes as a result of the material things they get in life. Are you falling into this trap? The truth is nothing outside can really make you happy. That is an illusion or a dream. The illusion is so strong that most of us believe it. But please don't take my word for this, think about your own experience and if you are not happy or if you are depressed then ask yourself why you are unhappy or depressed, is it because you think you need to have something?

"One in four of us will have a mental illness at some point. That is a lot of people."

--Alastair Campbell--

TALK WITH COUNSELOR/CASE MANAGER

As was previously stated, it's never too late to seek help for depression; it's been suggested to face the problem at the beginning of the symptoms. Seeking help for depression shows a great deal of strength and talking with your health care professional can also help you feel better. Psychotherapy is a general term that describes a form a treatment conducted by a mental health professional that is based on discussing and expressing feelings. Also, group therapy can be helpful because you are able to get feedback from people who are going through similar issues as you, and some people believe there is power in numbers. These types of therapy can choose to focus on the problems of the group or on the individual if necessary. They try to be more structured in nature but it really depends on what is going on in the group for that session. The structured approach to group therapy focuses on addressing attitudes and behaviors that contribute to depression but sometimes you may have someone who wants to share and work on more and that's ok. Your case manager can support people with depression by helping them find ways of effectively managing the situations that trigger the depression. These may include family issues, financial problems, work stress and living arrangements. Mental health social workers can also provide focused psychological self-help strategies, which include relaxation training and skills training.

Also, study has shown, talking about your thoughts and feelings with supportive person makes you feel better. It can be very healing to voice your worries or talk about something that's weighting on your mind. And it feels good to be listened to knowing that someone else cares about you and wants to help. It can be very helpful to talk about your problems to close friends and family members. But sometimes, we need help that the people around us aren't able to provide.

When you need extra support an outside perspective, or some expert guidance, talking to a therapist or counselor can help. While the support of friends and family is important, therapy is different. Therapists are professionally trained listeners who can help you get to the root of your problems, overcome emotional challenges, and make positive changes in your life. You don't have to be diagnosed with a mental health problem to benefit from therapy. Many people in therapy seek help for everyday concerns such as relationship problems, job stress, or self-doubt, or others turn to therapy during difficult times, such as a divorce.

"Mental illness, of course, is not literally a 'thing' - or physical object - and hence it can 'exist' only in the same sort of way in which other theoretical concepts exist."

--Thomas Szasz--

Chapter 3

HEARING VOICES
(Auditory Hallucinations)

Hearing voices is a common type of auditory hallucination; According to the National Institute of Mental Health NIMH, hallucinations are sensations or perceptions that occur in a wakeful state and seem real, but are created by the brain. The voices in auditory hallucinations can be pleasant or threatening. Doctors believe hearing voices can be associated with some psychiatric disorders or medical conditions. Some psychiatric conditions associated with hearing voices include bipolar disorder, psychotic depression, schizoid and schizotpal personality disorders, and schizophrenia says the NIMH. Also, auditory hallucinations can occur during medical conditions affecting the central nervous system such as brain tumors, delirium, dementia, epilepsy and other seizure disorders, and stroke, all of the above can be associated with hearing voices. It's been suggested voices may also be associated with high fevers.

In addition, some people say when they abuse certain substances it will cause them to hear voices because those substances can cause hallucinations, including hearing voices. Auditory and other hallucinations can also be associated with other substances, such as alcohol, when used in large quantities or during withdrawal says the National Institute of Mental Health. Also, hearing voices can also be a side effect of some medications and may occur with hearing loss, sleep deprivation, or sever fatigue. The specific cause of hallucinations, including hearing voices, is not known.

As a final point, hearing voices can be a symptom of serious and even life threatening, conditions. If you are experiencing auditory hallucinations (hearing voices) seek immediate medical care (call 911). Doctors suggest if you cannot distinguish the voices from reality or if the voices are accompanied by coloration of the lips or fingernails; chest pain or pressure, cold, clammy or dry, hot skin, confusion or loss of consciousness for even a moment, or high fever (higher than 101 degrees Fahrenheit) seek immediate medical care especially if the voices you hear are telling you to harm yourself or other. Seek prompt medical care if your being treated for a condition associated with hearing voices and your symptoms are constantly worsen, or otherwise cause you concern says Lloyd, Arthur of Hearing Voices.

DISTRACTIONS

A good way most people cope with distressing voices is distractions. Distractions will help you focus your mind on something else and you will forget or not notice what the voices are saying. For example, try going for a picnic with someone that will help you forget about what is on your mind. Or listen to energetic music; look over your gratitude list or create a list of good things you achieved and your assists or strengths. You can also look at photo albums of fun vacations and think of the good things others have said about you. Other examples, you can make yourself an emergency comfort bundle (of goodies) such as a good book, love letters, love poems, read joke books or a nice email you received or sent; say positive statements to yourself and record your positive statements on tape (your voice) and listen to them later, watch films that are comedy or inspirational. Still, it is possible we can be distracted and not experience mental illness. However, distractions can help or hinder you depending on how and when it enters your life. Namely, a loud noise, unruly children or a sudden rainstorm are all events that can distract us from what we're doing at the moment as well as hinder you. In all honesty, repetitive distraction, such as a nonstop ringing phones, incessant email and text message interruptions, meeting and co-workers who need immediate attention, can contribute to mental distress or even mental illness. When we are in the midst of a crisis where no immediate action needed. For example, when the death of a loved one occur, we may try distracting oneself from the emotional pain by taking a walk, reading a book or watching a movie to help us get through a painful situation.

Study has shown distraction is a helpful technique used for the treatment of depression, substance use and some compulsive behaviors.

In addition, researcher has discovered what happens when we switch our attention between multiple tasks. It's been said people with a higher caffeine intake, from sources such as coffee, tea, and caffeinated energy drinks, are more likely to report hallucinatory experiences such as hearing voices and seeing things that are not there.

Also, experts believe when under stress the body releases a stress hormone called cortisol, and more of this stress hormone is released in response to stress when people have recently had caffeine. It is this extra boost of cortisol which may link caffeine intake with an increased tendency to hallucinate, said the researchers. This isn't likely a concern for most people, as most people don't consume 7 or more cups of coffee every day. But it has a direct impact on people who might already be at greater risk for hearing voices or seeing things for instance, people with schizophrenia. People with schizophrenia who also drink large amounts of caffeine may be accidentally setting themselves up for greater risk for future hallucinations. So lay off the caffeine.

"Mental illness can happen to anybody. You can be a dustman, a politician, a Tesco worker…anyone. It could be your dad, your brother or your aunt."

--Frank Bruno--

EARPLUGS

According to National Institute of Mental Health (NIMH), not all people who hear voices will find a particular technique effective. For example, some of my clients found that wearing an earplug makes no difference whatsoever, while others will say it stop the voices, or help them cope, so I want to say it may help and it may not help. Many individuals find that the effectiveness of a particular technique wears off over time as the voices shift. And, you should remember that the voices may command you to stop using a particular technique or forbid you to try it because subconsciously you know it will help. For most people who hear voices, talking to others reduces the intrusiveness or even stops the voices completely. Also, being around friendly faces and spending time with people while wearing earplugs can be very effective at pushing voices into the background as well. If you know a person who is clearly distressed by voices and unable to discuss this with you, you should try to get them to use earplugs.

On the whole, researchers have documented, wearing an earplug in one ear has been shown to be helpful to many people who hear voices. It can reduce voice activity by nearly 50 per cent. It's been said that earplugs work in different ears for different people so try to switch ears to see which ear is more effective for you. By wearing one earplug rather than wearing two, the person is able to continue with normal social activities such as being able to hear other people, or the telephone. For example, some people find that the earplug seem to become less effective as a technique after some time has pass. Another difficulty is that the earplugs may be uncomfortable, or the person feels self conscious using one in public. However, earplugs work well for people who voices are particularly troublesome at night says voice hearers. You can use earplugs in either the right or left ear; though it seems for many people using a single earplug in the right ear works best.

It's been said the formal term describing this method is known as MONO-AURAL OCCLUSION (the word aural referring to the ear). For some people cotton wool plugs work but according to most people wear earplugs that can be molded to the inside of your ear (but don't push too hard) are generally the best. The wax earplugs generally have cotton wool mixed in them so there is no danger of them melting into your ear. It is suggested to try first the right ear for a period of time (say for two hours) and then again on the same ear later for the same period of time. Later on you can try the same with the left ear but on the different day. The main point is to use the earplugs for a limited period of time and only when the voices are at their worst or most loud.

"For too long we have swept the problems of mental illness under the carpet... and hoped that they would go away."

--Richard J. Codey--

THINKING (COGNITIVE APPROACH)

Thinking (termed cognitive) strategies means using your thoughts as a self aware way to challenge your thoughts or in some ways reduce the impact of the sense of the power that you may feel the voices have over you. The voices may be saying something about your friend or partner, and providing they are understanding and are not likely to take offence, you can nicely check with those people to see if what the voices have said about what they may be thinking is true. You can rest assure in the fact that generally the voices (I mean those of auditory hallucinations) have been found by the majority of voices hearers to be mostly unreliable, mischievous, or hazardous with regard to some of what they are proposing to you. You also have to be caution about the content of what you wish to check out with the person the voices are speaking about, because some of it may just be too intrusive or personal and may actually cause the other person to get offended. Remember, it may be the voices just want to get you into trouble or bring trouble in your friendships or with the people the voices are attacking.

In addition, psychological therapy professional believe negotiating (time out) with the voices or otherwise postponing (delaying) listening to the voices; in exchange for giving the voices your positive attention say for a half hour or an hour you ask them to go away for half or a whole day. You may have to experiment with this awhile to get some effect. It's like saying I will reward you with positive attention for a while by saying, if you will then shut-up for the next four hours or so. Or you say, if you go away now I will give positive attention towards the end of the day say 5pm etc. If you don't feel too frightened of the voices you could practice dismissing them; it's been reported that this can really work for some people and build up their confidence over controlling some of the voices.

It's been reported that telling the voices to go away in a firm manner can sometimes cause them to go for awhile. A variation of the above method would be for you to just tell the voices to shut up and on doing so, IMMEDIATELY DIVDERT YOURSELF onto a distraction or concentration activity: even if the voices still stay around, continue to ignore them for a contain period of time before giving them any attention. Psychological therapy professional calls this technique, "thought stopping" it is often listen and described in certain books as psychological therapies. Some people find actively ignoring the voices can be effective for getting them to go for a while. It is said, it is generally easier to do this by doing some other activity.

"Negative attitudes will never result in a positive life!"
--Ema White--

CONCENTRATION

Concentration is a technique most people use to help drown out voices. Some example of things you can do to improve your concentration are reading, studying, writing a journal or dairy, or learning creative writing such as for a story, play, poem or maybe doing proof reading on someone else's work: or it might be doing art work or sculpting or something related. Please note that studying is not recommended for those people who might for example get badly stressed by this activity due to past negative experiences. It's a fact that some people can be tripped into an episode of mental distress or even illness just from the pressures of studying. The pressure of studying for and exam may just act as the trigger for illness which may have had other contributory factors in that person's background; that's why most people in college take a leave of absence if they are having serious mental health issues until they feel they are ready to handle deadlines and homework. Instead of studying you could include putting together model airplanes, jigsaw puzzles, undertaking DIY or repairing things at home or maybe at someone else's place.

In addition, you can try playing or learning chess; shoot pool, go to a bowling alley, play racket sports. Or it could be playing a musical instrument e.g. guitar, drum, violin or keyboard instrument synthesizer. Moreover, it could be things like singing specific tunes or songs, even attending a choir etc. Plus, it might include certain types of physical exercises, like working out at the Gym, Yoga, or swimming. Try to do specific tasks in your head that you might otherwise use your mouth. An example of this method would be counting (in your head up to 100 rather than aloud) or reciting a poem in your head or the words of a song that you like. It's been suggested to develop a coping method chart to record the different types of coping skills that you use.

Using this chart will help you experiment or try out the different coping methods so that the results of your success can be remembered more easily. You can then use the charts to make a short list of the coping methods that work best for you.

> *"Whenever I write about mental health and integrative therapies, I am accused of being prejudice against pharmaceuticals. So let me be clear-integrative medicine is the judicious application of both conventional and evidence-based natural therapies."*
>
> *--Andrew Weil--*

RELAXATION

As I stated previously in this book, listening to a relaxation tape involves auditory stimulation and distraction as well as encourage you to concentrate on carrying out the exercises. Therefore, this reduces the anxiety and contributes to the reduction in the intensity of the auditory hallucinations. Many people who hear voices find them particularly problematic at night. Therefore, playing relaxing music or a relaxation tape at bedtime can be helpful. Try these relaxation strategies that is suggest to help you sleep at night.

Give yourself permission to relax.

Recognize and acknowledge fears, then consciously let go of them.

Prayer/Meditation

Massage/acupuncture/yoga

Focus on your breathing/breathe deeply.

Listen to guided relaxation CDs.

Listen to soothing music.

Relax each muscle individually.

Self-Care and Comfort/Keep a list of achievements and strengths or a list of positive things other people have said about you.

Positive self-talk and self-forgiveness.

Look at comforting items e.g. e-mails, love letters, birthday cards, and photos.

Take a warm, scented bath. Wear comfortable clothes.

Get help with practical problems e.g. housing, finances.

Remember that situation/feelings frequently change-"this too shall pass."

Record positive statements onto a CD so you can listen to it later.

Eat a healthy diet. Do something nice for yourself each day.

Keep in frequent contact with support network, even if feeling okay.

Buy/pick fresh flowers. Change the sheets on your bed Get a pet, or help care for someone else's. Hold a safe, comforting object.

Holidays Humor/ Plan the day to ensure there aren't long periods of time with nothing to do.

"Exercise keeps me occupied, which is good for my mental health."

--Gail Porter—

TALKING

Talking in general helps people with mental health illness and for most people who hear voices talking reduces the intrusiveness or even stops the voices. Being around friendly faces and spending time with people can be very effective at pushing voices into the background. This is why when people troubled by voices (in the hospital) they seek out nurses or fellow patients to talk to, according to National Institute of Mental Health (NIMH) this is said to be a coping strategy. If a person is clearly distressed by voices and unable to discuss what he/she is going through, a nurse could try approaching the individual and talking to him/her. The reasons why social contact helps a person hearing voices may be difficult to explain but, many factors are involved, including distraction, vocalization and reassurance from the presence of others. Also, you might take time to speak with a partner, a close friend, or even a sympathetic worker, if you for example live in some kind of formal residential setting. You can telephone a friend or relative who are fairly supportive to you even they may not necessarily understand your experience. Or you can attend groups, such as peer support groups (one for voice hearers if possible), or join a hobby/activity groups.

Also, some people can find being among loving or supportive friends or in a caring relationship does not always make them feel more at ease, sometime people can feel worse: this can be related to their own personal feelings of low self esteem, or feeling they've let themselves or others down, it can also come from uncomfortable feelings produced by comparing of where one is, in relation to other peers you perceive as being more successful than yourself. It is important to avoid gatherings where you may feel too watched or too crowed in.

And, equally important unless duty calls for this avoid staying too long in the presence of people you perceive as being negatively critical as opposed to constructively critical because this can lead to an increase in both stress and by association the intensity of the voices. People who hear voices can also experience the sense that other people can read their mind say NIMH. Bear in mind the evidence for real telepathy suggest this is rather more limited than people often imagine. However, some people do find being on their own is more comfortable than being in the company of others. It's been said being in company of people particularly like public transportation can bring on more stress or worsen the voices.

"I try to make my bed every day for mental health. Coming home to an unmade bed or a room with clothes all over will depress me."

--David Alan Grier--

REMIND YOURSELF IT'S NOT REAL

According to the Mental Health Foundation, hearing voices in your head is often a sign of mental medical issues. Sometimes, the voices actually seem like an auditory voice, but there is just no one standing there. Other times, the voices seem like they are actually in the head, some even feel like the voices are in other body parts. It often occurs to people who have recently lost loved ones. It is considered an auditory hallucination. It is important to speak with a counselor or therapist or other people who hear voices to see how to handle the experience. Sound research with many voice hearers, both within and outside of mental health services, has found that voice hearers cope with their voices (or don't) depends not on the content of the voice experience (which can be either abusive and devaluing or guiding and inspiring or both) but on the nature of the relationship with the voices.

In addition, if you believe the voices are in control of you then you can't cope or if you believe you are stronger than the voices are, you can. This means it is no longer a sustainable position to think of voices as part of a disease syndrome, such as schizophrenia. Experts believe, hearing voices can be regarded as a meaningful, real (although sometimes painful, fearful and overwhelming) experience that speak to the person in a metaphorical way about their life, emotions and environment. For instance, people experiencing distress as a consequence of abusive or commanding voices can often recognize their voices as those of their actual abusers and the voices have the effect of attacking their sense of self esteem and worth says the mental Health Foundation.

Note: If you believe in God, if you hear someone claiming to be "God" talking to you and "he" tells you to harm another person or yourself, seek help from the psychiatrist or psychologist or call 911.

"The mental health conversation is very important to me. I have friends that struggle with various mental illnesses. I've struggled with depression and anxiety. I'm very interested in how we deal with that."

--Matthew quick--

TALK TO OTHER VOICE HEARERS

Talking to other voices hearers gives you the opportunity to share experiences and to learn from one another. Voice hearers say it's important to discuss their voices because this helps you learn to recognize their games and tricks, as well as their good aspects, and to identify patterns that are specific to given situations. Voice hearers may think they are alone in hearing voices (as most people with mental illness). This can lead to feelings of shame or the fear of going mad. According to voice hearer they feel they have the need to seek explanations to account for their voices and understand where the voices come from and why. What triggers them can be helpful in developing a coping strategy. Also, it's been said sharing experiences enables voice hearers to get to know what medicines others are using, how useful these are, and what their side effects may be. It is important, for example, to know whether a particular medicine is helpful in reducing the hearing of voices or easing anxiety and confusion. Although medication effects people in a different way, it will be helpful for you to know what others are taking and what the side-effects are. This information will help you to make a decision on what you should do for yourself.

Moreover, sharing knowledge about voices with families and friends can be helpful. If family and friend can understand the voices they can be more supportive. This can make voices hearer lives easier and improve their confidence in social situations. Individuals, who learned to adjust to their experiences, reported that the process has contributed to their personal growth. Personal growth can be defined as recognizing what you need in order to live a "normal" and fulfilled life, and knowing how to achieve it. It is important to recognize the wide variety of individual situations and circumstances as well.

According to the Mental Health Foundation, the best advices are to try to increase your influences over your voices, rather than intensify their powerlessness. It is recommended to avoid, places or situations where there is a lot of un-patterned background noise such as busy roads, or places where there is a lot of background noise, as these may increase the intensity of voices. And as I stated before, try to dismiss the voices, some people find that firmly telling the voices to stop or that they will be attended to latter provides some relief.

"Everyone says to you, 'if you play Ophelia, you'll end up crazy,' but we're all somewhere on the spectrum of mental health, and I think that if you approach it that way it's not such an intimidating issue."
--Guru Mbathe-Raw--

FOCUSING

It's been said, focusing will help you identify if the voices have a pattern. This can be a useful step because it gives you information about the behavior of the voices. Knowing the pattern of the voices may give you ideas on how you might deal with them. One advantage of using focusing when you hear voices is it gives you the opportunity to take a step back from the voices. And, is a way of using thinking about the voices in a more structured way. It is said it is generally easier for people to talk about the behavior of the voices rather than about what the voices is actually saying. According National Institute of Mental Health, most if not all voices will have a pattern of appearing and disappearing; or if not then of increasing or diminishing in loudness and frequency. This is often related to stress triggers; either a single big event (or a collection of lesser events) that produce, anxiety, fear, upset or worries. It's been suggested, to help to work this pattern out you need to keep a simply diary (or use a calendar) and mark out the days when your voices are worst. A detailed way of recording the activity of the voices is to score them out of ten. Below 4 the voices are of low or slight irritation, scores of 4-6, means they are affecting concentration, at 7 upwards means they are a serious distraction.

To add, you could create your own simple hand drawn graph or use the graphs you get on fairly cheap arithmetic exercise books bought from your local store. The upwards (vertically drawn) is divided either into 7 days or more. On this kind of scale 0 means no voices whatsoever, 10 means voices are continuous from the time you're awake to the time you have gone to sleep. Recording or checking out the pattern of your voices can be regarded as a form of coping. You are using your time to check them out to see if they have a pattern of coming and going.

Actually seeing that they do have a pattern of coming and going does two things: One, the fact they have a pattern makes them a bit less mysterious; and two, if you are able to relate to their pattern of coming and going to events in your life you will be able to opens up the possibility of having some control over the voices. That is if you can see how the stress triggers your voices; it follows that it might be possible to work out ways in which you could either reduce the number of stress triggers affecting you or better still to reduce the way those triggers impact you says NIMH.

Lastly, focusing is not in itself a quick fix for the annoyance of the voices. The value of such knowledge may be more helpful with coping with the voices in the long term; so any knowledge you get of their pattern is generally not wasted and can be used to experiment with how you reduce or simply deal with the stress events that form and triggers your voices. People can use this technique by themselves, but it is often better to do this with a worker or someone who can stand outside of your situation and who wants to help you.

"I can understand why some people might look at me and say, 'What's she got to be depressed about?' I get that a lot in Britain, where mental health issues seem to be a big taboo."
--Natalie Lmbruglia--

MEDICATION

According to, National Institute of Mental Health, alcohol, cannabis, crack cocaine and amphetamines are sometimes use when an individual wants to self medicate. These substances might not always start the problem but, it appears to bring short term relief. But, in the long run it will always make the voices worse. Additionally such substance will often have other unpleasant effects which in the long term usually impair physical health. Use of these substance alongside the medication, either neutralizes the beneficial effects of the medication or strengthens certain affects. For example like making people even more sleepy, depressed or worse more paranoid and apt to misinterpret what might be going around them. It is helpful to acknowledge that some voices hearer may not always find medications given for their voices to be effective or perhaps feel the side effects of the medication to be as bad as or worse than the annoyance of their voices. In fact, research shows that between 25%-40% of people on medication still hear voices. This does not mean that the medications should be discontinued it just means you should carefully weigh other benefits and take the hazards into account before any decision is taken to continue or discontinue them. Such as those of increasing sleep, improving mood etc, may still be valuable enough to make them worth taking once the balance of risks are carefully discussed with your Doctor, other professional worker or advocate.

In addition, all medications prescribed by Doctors to help relieve the voices needs to be carefully supervised or monitored because of the very distressing side effects that might occur. Such as, weight gain, depression, loss of libido or impotence, sensitivity to sun burn, occasionally breast enlargement in males, stiffness (Parkinson like symptoms), heavy salivation, or unpleasant involuntary twitching or muscles or worse dramatic involuntary movements of legs, mouth tongue muscle says NIMH. Also, experts believe such medications may effects the production of certain blood cells, so it is very important to try to read any leaflets on side effects or to get someone else to read and explain it to you especially if you suffer blurring of vision. There are also various books on this topic. Keep in mind such books do tend to get out of date fairly quickly as new medications hit the market while even more recent research on the previous ones comes out.

> "As the national Football League and other pro sports increasingly reckon with the early dementia, mental health issues, suicides and even criminal behavior of former players, the risk of what's known as chronic traumatic encephalopathy (CTE), is becoming clear."
>
> *--Jeffrey Kluger--*

Chapter 4

DRUGS AND ALCOHOL

As you know an addiction to drugs or alcohol can affect every aspect of your life. It can cause financial problems, relationship problems, mental health problems, and health problems. Drugs and alcohol cause you to act in ways that you would never even consider under normal circumstances. Addiction not only puts you in danger, but may also put those you love in danger as well. The facts show there are many drugs that can cause addiction. These include marijuana, heroin, cocaine, crack cocaine, methamphetamines and some prescription drugs. Each drug cause a different reaction, but they all impair your ability to think rationally and clearly. It's been said drug addiction causes you to continually use more and more to get the feeling you are trying to achieve. Addiction to drugs can cause many different health problems, including stroke, cardiovascular disease, lung problems, cancer and mental disorders says the Alcoholism Guide to Recovery (AGR). There are several kinds of alcohol, the alcohol that people drink as called ethanol, which is a sedative. When you consume alcohol it is absorbed into the bloodstream and affects the nervous system. It blocks messages from reaching the brain, causing impairment to your vision, perception, emotions and movement.

Also, alcohol abuse is a prolonged drinking habit that can cause problems in other areas of your life. It has be said, long term alcohol use can cause significant health problems, including liver problems, heart problems, memory loss, skin problems and damage to your nervous system says AGR.

In addition, some of the visible signs that someone is abusing drugs or alcohol are the abuse of it. Some signs that you or someone you know is abusing are regular use of drugs and alcohol, lying about how often they use, avoiding friends and family, using drugs and alcohol alone, giving up sports or activities that they have always done, and constantly talking about drugs or alcohol. Also, they may have a drastic change in personality. Other signs such as being abnormally moody, agitated, irritated may also signal an addiction. Some treatment options are rehabilitation centers for those addicted to drugs or alcohol. Some programs require extended stay inside the treatment facility, while others offer outpatient treatment. Determining the best treatment will depend on what you are addicted to, how long you have been using the drug or alcohol, and if there are any medical problems that would complicate the treatment. After you are off the drugs or alcohol, you may still need some form of treatment for the rest of your life says National Institute on Alcohol Abuse and Alcoholism.

Warning: The abuse of drugs or alcohol can be dangerous. Consuming too much alcohol can cause alcohol poisoning and can result in death; taking too much drugs can cause an overdose, which can result in death. Driving or operating other machinery can lead to accidents that can result in your death or the death or other people, says The National Institute on Alcohol Abuse and Alcoholism.

ALCOHOL USE AND ABUSE: WHAT YOU SHOULD KNOW

For some people drinking alcoholic beverages is often seen as a way to relax, socialize or celebrate, but drinking too much or drinking as a way of dealing with feelings of anxiety or depression has negative consequences. The amount of liquid that is consumed (a drink) depends on the type of alcohol being consumed. The National Institute on Alcohol Abuse and Alcoholism (NIAAA) defines the following as one standard drink. One, it is advised that men consume no more than 3 drinks in a single day or 7 drinks total in a week, this is only a rough guidelines; pregnant women, people under the age of 21 or people with health conditions or medications that interact with alcohol should not drink alcohol. Alcohol has many short and long term effects. In the short term, it's been said after changes in mood and decreased inhibition have passed, one may experience a hangover. Hangovers often described as feelings of dehydration, a sense of mental fogginess, headache and nausea. In the long term, heavy alcohol use can lead to serious organ damage and memory problems. In addition, here are some other effects of alcohol that you may not be as familiar with: According to the NIAAA, while alcohol may cause some people to be able to fall asleep more quickly, it decreases the quality of sleep by interfering with REM 3 REM (rapid eye movement) which is a part of the sleep cycle when dreams occur, and is thought to be the most healing stage of sleep. If REM sleep is disrupted you may feel tired and unable to concentrate the next day. Also, it is said alcohol alters serotonin levels in the brain. Serotonin is a neurotransmitter, or chemical, used by the brain to regulate mood, and imbalances. Serotonin is said to cause mental health conditions like depression, anxiety and obsessive compulsive disorder.

In addition, it's been suggested, a heavy drinker is when someone consumes more than the daily or weekly guideline amounts for alcohol. Binge Drinking is when excessive amounts of alcohol are consumed in a short period of time, resulting in a spike in blood alcohol content (a man who has 5 drinks in 2 hours, or a women who has 4 drinks during that time) people who binge drink are especially prone to "blackouts" or lapses in memory says NIAAA. Alcoholism, also known as alcohol dependence, is a disorder characterized by an uncontrollable urge to drink, inability to stop drinking once started, need to drink more and more to feel the effects (tolerance), and withdrawal symptoms if one does not consume alcohol. Doctors reported withdrawal symptoms can include anxiety, sweating, nausea or shaking. If you need help dealing with your drinking or drug use, try contacting your employer's employee assistance program (EAP) and/or primary care doctor.

"My worst days in recovery are better than the best days in relapse."

--Kate Le Page--

ATTEND ALCOHOLIC ANNONYMOUS (AA)

Alcoholics Anonymous is said to be a "fellowship of men and women who share their experience, strength and hope with each other that they may solve their common problem and help others to recover from alcoholism." The only requirement for membership is a desire to stop drinking. There are no dues or fee for AA membership, they are self supporting through their own contributions. AA is not connected with any denomination, politics, organization or institution, and does not wish to engage in any controversy, nether endorses nor opposes any cause. Their primary purpose is to stay sober and help other alcoholics to achieve sobriety says AA. Alcoholics Anonymous, usually abbreviated AA, is a 12-step recovery program that has helped many people stop the use of alcohol. The original program was focused on spirituality, religion, and God having an impact on changing a person's life, but depending on the program you attend, these 12 steps may be altered for the audience. AA is completely confidential, and it is assumed that all participants will remain anonymous. No participant is supposed to discuss others outside the group, and this is for safety and reputation's sake. Participants are usually told to accept a sponsor from the group. This is a person who has already successfully passed though the program. The person will act as a focus for support and will help the participant through the stages of the program. We will talk more about sponsors in another chapter.

The A.A. Preamble: "Alcoholics Anonymous is a fellowship of men and women who share their experience, strength and hope with each other that they may solve their common problem and help others to recover from alcoholism." The only requirement for membership is a desire to stop drinking. There are no dues or fees for A.A. membership; they are Self-supporting through their own contributions.

"A.A. is not allied with any sect, denomination, politics, organization or institution; does not wish to engage in any controversy; neither endorses nor opposes any causes." Their primary purpose is to stay sober and help other alcoholics to achieve sobriety (AA). AA has helped many people in my group achieve sobriety.

"Mania starts off fun, not sleeping for days, keeping company with your brain, which has become a wonderful computer, showing 24 TV channels all about you. That goes horribly wrong after awhile."

--Carrier Fisher--

DETOXIFICATION PROGRAM

One of the benefits of a detox program is that your personal treatment plan can be customized to suit your specific situation because every person has different needs. For example, the facts show a drug detox program may be based on the amount and types of drugs you are currently using. This is an important point because opiate detoxification can be quite different from alcohol detoxification. Your personalized detox program may also be designed to include other factors such as relevant medical or psychological conditions, says the Alcoholism Guide to Recovery (AGR). Moreover, a variety of other factors can be involved in designing an individualized detox program, including your own motivation in terms of completing the program successfully. According to AGR, the first goal of a detox facility is to help you gently expel any toxins from your body. So the sooner you choose a detox facility, the better your opportunity to achieve long term recovery will be. Weather you need a facility that caters toward opiate detoxification or some other type of substance detox, this is the first step. It is never too late to begin a fresh new start on life. So get started. According to treatment centers, there is other effective alternative treatment for alcoholism which include Nutritional therapy. Most alcoholics suffer from a lack of nutrients, as well as liver damage from years of substance abuse. Other treatment centers, goes on to say to reduce craving from alcohol, repair the body of its lost nutrients. Zinc and vitamin C help with the detoxification process, as the body is full of toxins at this point in the treatment. Vitamin B is essential, especially thiamine (B1). Thiamine reduces a person's alcohol cravings and is barely existent in an alcoholic. A strict diet would be prescribed and used to regulate blood sugar and balance the body, eventually leading to the elimination of alcohol cravings.

Also, herbal therapy can go hand-in-hand with nutritional therapy; specific herbs can be administered to ease the detoxification process. It's been suggested, chamomile, peppermint and skullcap can be made into a tea to calm the mind when anxiety hits. ST. John's wort can help with depression and unease. Kudzu root, in the form of a tea, is used in Chinese medicine to help reduce the craving for alcohol. Turmeric and milk thistle are known to clean the blood and help purify the liver. In addition, acupuncture is the ancient Chinese medicinal practice of manipulating pressure points throughout the body with tine needles.

It has been known to cure chemical dependency, depression and detoxification. Try starting a meditation program because addiction is more than physical. In order to be successful in your recovery, you need to look within yourself for the root cause of your pain. Through meditation, you can calm your mind and take responsibility for your actions. Eventually, and with practice, you can find peace and move on from troubled times. Using these alternative therapies in combination with one another is recommended to ensure success in your recovery. This is a long road; know that you are not alone.

"It's a bit like walking down a long, dark corridor never knowing when the light will go on."
--Neil Lennon—

REMOVE DRUG PARAPHERNALIA

This refers to removing all things that can trigger an alcohol addiction relapse. Alcohol dependence is an addiction like any other. True addictions are chronic conditions thus there is no permanent cure. There is always the potential for alcohol addiction relapse, so you must be careful to avoid situations that can trigger it.
If you have negative feelings often, especially low self esteem anger or resentment, it puts you at serious risk of alcohol addiction relapse. You may need to work with a professional therapist to learn how to deal with these issues. It may seem obvious, but too many former alcoholics don't take this seriously, being around other who is drinking can definitely trigger a relapse, especially if they are consuming excessively and are having a good time. Try to avoid situations where other are drinking around you, and if you must be around alcohol, ask someone who doesn't drink to go with you for support.

In addition, ask yourself does looking at a hand pipe, bottle of alcohol, or rolling papers trigger the need to get high in a person that like to get stone? That's the consensus of a new study that finds drug paraphernalia has the power to activate reward center in the brains of marijuana users and produce a need for weed. Researchers from the University of Texas at Dallas recently published this research in the late edition of the journal Drug and Alcohol Dependence, which indicates the brains of drug user and those of sober society react differently when subjected to paraphernalia stimuli. While the National Institute on Drug Abuse claims that cannabis has a nine percent addiction rate, the federal agency fails to mention that weed is no more of a detriment than caffeine, which has the same risk for dependence.

Researchers say marijuana activates similar areas of the brain that are often triggered by highly addictive substances like nicotine and cocaine, Incidentally, what they fail to mention is that the reward centers in the brain can also be triggered by the anticipation of good food. "Like addictive drugs, highly palatable foods trigger feel-good brain chemical such as dopamine says the National Institute on Drug Abuse.

"The lows were absolutely horrible. It was like falling into a manhole and not being able to lift the lid and climb out."
--Linda Hamilton--

REPLACING ADDICTIONS WITH A HEALTHY OBSESSIONS

According to Dr. Lance Dodes, assistant clinical professor of psychiatry at Harvard Medical School and the author of Breaking Addiction, many recovering addicts simply transfer from one obsession to another. "It's been well known for a very long time that A.A. meeting used to be filled with smoke because people shifted their focus from drinking to cigarettes, "he says. "Alcoholism isn't about alcohol any more than compulsive gambling is about playing roulette or winning money. Addiction is a solution to an emotional need. If you deprive someone of one solution to their emotional problems, it's not surprising that they'll find another one instead." Dr. Harold Urschel, chief medical strategist of Inter-health Addiction Disease Management Company and the author of Healing the Addicted Brain, says that untreated psychiatric disorders may also drive recovering addicts to new compulsions, "you may get sober but all of a sudden, you realize you have an anxiety disorder or depression, "he says. "You may go get on porn sites because it help reduce your anxiety or go gambling because when you hit the jackpot, it feels really good and helps lift your depression."

In addition, in 2008 the National Institute on Drug abuse pledged $4 million dollars to research the effect of physical activity on drug use. Preclinical research was provided evidence that exercise, can help treat, and even possibly prevent addiction, and now human trials are taking place. "Habits play an important role in our health", the institute's director, Dr. Nora Volkow, said in a National Institute of Healthy newsletter. "Understanding the biology of how we develop routines that may be harmful to us, and how to break those routines and embrace new ones, could help us change our lifestyles and adopt healthier behaviors."

The facts show, exercise and sporting groups could help fill that void, said Richard Brown, a professor of psychiatry and human behavior at Brown University and director of addictions research at Butler Hospital in Providence, Rhode Island. When Brown and his colleagues started their human study on exercise and alcohol abuse, they theorized that physical activity would reduce the depressive symptoms alcoholics often suffer from thereby reducing the risk of a relapse. What the researchers didn't expect was the feedback from participants who said they enjoyed replacing their addiction with exercising because it provided the structure that was needed in their lives.

"Mental illness is an equal-opportunity illness. Every one of us is impacted by mental illness. One in five adults is dealing with this illness, and many are not seeking help because the stigma prevents that."

--Margaret Larson—

PRAYER

To put it briefly, it is not a good idea to replace medical treatments with prayer. Some people do have such a strong faith in prayer that they are willing to rely on it completely. Those people who have an addictive personality have tendency for overdoing things. Prayer can be a wonderful addiction to a person's life so long as they do not use it as a means to escape reality. To add, Alcoholics Anonymous, (AA) has serenity prayer for most individuals who attend meetings. One Way of defining serenity is to say that it is a feeling of being calm and tranquil. In recovery this word is often used to describe a state of being where people are untroubled by the ups and downs in life. It means that whatever is happening in the individual's life they can rely on an inner sense of calm. Many would say that this way of being is the goal of recovery. It may even have been the search for such inner peace that drove the individual into addiction in the first place. Most people find what they are looking for in sobriety.

On the other hand, Thomas Szasz provides another way of looking at serenity with his words: "Boredom is the feeling that everything is a waste of time; serenity that nothing is." The serenity prayer was created in 1937 by a theologian called Karl Paul Reinhold Niebuhr. The original text for this prayer was. "Father, give us courage to change what must be altered, serenity to accept what cannot be helped, and the insight to know the one from the other. A slightly different version of the prayer has been adopted by 12 step group which is God grant me the serenity to accept the things I cannot change, courage to change the things I can change, and wisdom to know the difference. In addition, they also have a Serenity Prayer for Non Believers: For some people, the word God and prayer can make non believers feel uncomfortable.

This might lead them to conclude that the serenity prayer has nothing to offer them. In fact there is a great deal that these words can offer the non believer without them needing to adopt any religious ideas. They can view God as nature or their own inner wisdom. The important thing to remember is it's not the actual words used but the sentiment which each individual can interpret in their own way.

Here are 10 reasons AA suggest why the Serenity Prayer can benefit everyone in recovery.

- 1. Acceptance as the Key to Happiness
- 2. The serenity prayer gives comfort when times are hard
- 3. It develop faith in recovery
- 4. It takes courage to build a new life
- 5. Gain importance of becoming wise in recovery
- 6. Serenity means developing equanimity
- 7. The serenity prayer empowers the individual
- 8. Increased contact with the spiritual path
- 9. Serenity power and positive thinking
- 10. Serenity prayer laid foundation of humility

"You have good days and bad days, and depressions something that, you know, is always with you."
--Winona Ryder--

(AA) BIG BOOK

The Big book is Alcoholics Anonymous (AA) inspirational books for people in recovery. Most people feel books can help them stay sober, just relying on books alone will not be enough to keep you sober, but reading the right material can certainly help. There are now thousands of titles that will be available on the interest to people recovering from addiction. These books contain valuable information and inspiring stories. Reading such material will keep people motivated so that they can build a good life in recovery. It is recommended that those in early recovery especially should immerse themselves in this recovery literature. It will help strengthen your determination and provide inspiration. Here are just a few of the most popular books that are currently available: Alcoholics Anonymous: The big book by Anonymous. When this book was originally released back in 1939 the original title was Alcoholics Anonymous: The story of how more than 100 men have recovered from alcoholism. It is now better known as the big book. Since publication, it has sold over 20 million copies, making it the most successful recovery book ever written. It contains a full explanation of the 12 step program, and sections of this book are routinely read at AA meetings. Anyone who intends to follow the AA method to help them stay sober should read this book. 12 Stupid Things That Mess Up Recovery: this book deals mostly with the issues that people are likely to face in early recovery.

To add, Dr Berger defined early recovery as the first two years in sobriety. His opinions are based on his years working as a clinician and his personal experience of dealing with addiction. Much of the material is influenced by the 12 step program, but there are insights that will be of use to anyone in recovery. This small book (128 pages) is packed with useful information.

Rational Recovery: The New Cure for Substance Addiction. Much of the popular recovery literature is based around 12 step programs. The new Cure for Substance Addiction offers a radically different approach. Other professional clinician disagrees with the A philosophy. Instead some offers a technique that involves learning to defend against the addictive voice. Those individuals who follow the Rational Recovery guidelines do not have to go to meetings for the rest of their life. All the information they need is in this book, though there is plenty of other related material available to buy. Those who use this method are not expected to keep referring to themselves as alcoholics. There is debate about the effectiveness of this approach, but it does seem to work for some people. Stage II Recovery: Life Beyond Addiction, this is useful read for people who are in their first 5 years of sobriety. It emphasizes the idea that recovery is a process and not an event. This book gives readers and idea of what to expect in recovery and prepares them for the challenges they are likely to face. As the title suggest the focus here is not on accepting addiction but on building a great life away from alcohol and drugs.

"I want to break down some of the stigma associated with mental illness."

--Gail Porter--

SPONSOR

In most organizations and social groups, a sponsor is someone who initially introduces you into the group and who vouches for your good character. This is not the case in Alcoholics Anonymous (AA). An AA sponsor is a person who has been abstinent for a long period and who is prepared to support a newly abstinent member. The sponsorship idea is a vital part of the Alcoholics Anonymous set up, and part of its social support network. It is all about social responsibilities, living up to them and doing one's duty to help each other. It is an unwritten rule of sponsorship that consists of choosing your own. If the person agree to sponsor you, but AA prefers them to be of the same sex, believing that mixed sex sponsor pairs cause unwanted complications (the idea that a man and woman cannot have a platonic relationship being part of this no doubt). It is not forbidden to have a sponsor of the opposite sex, but is not advised. You have to choose your sponsor wisely though as they become a very influential figure in your life, and a crutch in time of your greater need. Sponsors are at liberty to tell you that they cannot help if they have urgent business elsewhere. However, they have a moral duty to put you in contact with another reliable person if you are facing a crisis and possible alcoholism relapse and they cannot support you at that time

In addition, if you want to ask an AA member to sponsor you, my advice to you is to attend a number of meetings and just watch the members sharing. Focus on those who seem to be living good lives and are content. If they have what you want, chances are that they will make a good sponsor. There is no mad rush to find a sponsor, obviously if you keep putting it off that is not good. However, be sure of the person that you choose, ultimately they are going to help you stay sober so choosing well is important.

If after a short time you feel that you made the wrong choice then by all means find someone else. It's your life and it's your sobriety. Don't compromise it because you don't want to hurt the feelings of your sponsor. It can seem like the hardest thing in the world to ask an AA member to take you on as a sponsor. You might ask yourself, what if they say no. For most people this is a common barrier to asking somebody. So what if they say no, it's no reflection on you. There could be a thousand reasons as to why they refuse. Don't wonder about it look for somebody else. And remember always go for someone who's recovery inspires you.

"I promise you nothing is as chaotic as it seems. Nothing is worth your health. Nothing is worth poisoning yourself into stress, anxiety, and fear."

--Steve Maraboli—

BUILDING A RECOVERY SUPPORT GROUP

Alcohol Anonymous (AA) suggested these 3 steps on how to succeed in finding a reliable support group. First, you cannot do it on your own, remember every time you tried to quit and stay sober alone, it failed. Addiction is a disease of isolation and recovery is about connection with others. Second, find and utilize people who are successfully in long term recovery. Follow how those people are actually doing it not just talking the talk. This might affect you down the road because without friends, isolation can takeover, isolation and boredom are breeding grounds for addiction. Be sure and remember that there are millions in recovery and you could be one of them if you do what they do. Third, Try out a few different support groups (never put all your eggs in one basket). Experts believe some rules of addiction recovery are golden rules and should be taken into account forever instead of forgotten. These are useful and important trail markers to guide you and help you stay on the right track. Also, 12 step meetings have been found to be very effective for most people. Just about every treatment center recommends them as a foundation of your social support because they work. There are various reasons you should do this carefully because if the first meeting you go to doesn't suit your needs, you may give up on the entire idea of support groups instead of simply finding one to your liking. Make sure the professional support people in your life such as counselors and doctors know the whole story. Addiction causes changes in our body and mind; do not keep addiction history from them.

Also, enlist the support of your family but realize they cannot be your only support. Addiction is a family disease and they may have their own issues to work on such as anger, enabling or codependency.

You may accomplish this by opening communication with them and setting some limits and boundaries. You need to work on your issues and they need to work on theirs. They may help but you cannot take on their problems and try to solve them as well as your own. This may make a difference to you as it empowers your own recovery and is a method to keep you accountable.

Following these golden rules to develop a large social support network and you will probably find your life easier, your progress rapid as well as your successes more frequent. Addiction recovery can certainly be done with the aid and support of people around you. Alone, it is next to impossible.

"She who has hope has everything."
--Anonymous--

PEOPLE, PLACES, AND THINGS

Study has shown to help fight addiction cravings, it is often useful to identify under what circumstances craving occur. Cravings in your addiction can come from both positive events and negative events. They can be caused by people you're with, your location, or something you're doing. Cravings are intellectually ridiculous, but that doesn't stop the gut wrenching pull toward your old addictive behavior. Now ask yourself, do the alcoholic who is in recovery place themselves in situations where they are hanging around with their old drinking buddy who is an active alcoholic? No. but if so, then the chances is greater that they will start drinking again. Any time that the people around them are consuming alcoholic beverages, the person who used to struggle with drinking is at risks. Your old bunch of people you use to be with at the party don't have much respect for sober people. It is said that relapsing is always one drink away. It's just a wise decision to not place oneself in arms way. Breaking loose from an alcoholic spouse, friend or relative to ensure sobriety stays intact may be necessary but is hard for most people. It is very important to keep a safe distance from people who party a lot when you are recovering from alcohol. It is vitally important in the beginning of sobriety that you stay away from old habits by avoiding relationships with old friends. By doing this, the chances that a recovered alcoholic will drank again are lessened. As with anything else in your life the person who is sober must rub shoulders with like minded people.

To add, this is where organizations like Alcohol Anonymous (AA) come into play on how to change person, places or things. By attending alcoholism support group meeting regularly, a new way of life begins to form along with an entirely new bunch of friends. Letting go of old friends is not as easy as it sounds. It will take a lot of determination.

Your new friends will help keep you from relapsing if you stay in close contact with them. It should go without saying you will have to stay out of bars. If the place where the most alcohol used to be consumed is your job, then it's time to find a new job. Anything that can compel the recovering person to drink should be eliminated from their daily routine. If they continue to do what they have always done they will get what they have always gotten, "drunk. Lastly, in recovery an alcoholic learns that the most important thing to them must be staying sober.

Sometimes you may have to move into a small house to relieve the stress of having to work two jobs to pay the bills. Then that's what you do. If they have to get rid of a few things that would hinder you from attending support group meetings on a regular basis then get rid of them. In relation to things, if the sober person has difficulty with looking at their favorite brand of beer, wine or lacquer, then they should stay away from those isles or just don't watch TV for awhile.

"Hope is a renewable option: If you run out of it at the end of the day, you get to start over in the morning."
--Barbara Kingsolver--

Chapter 5

STRESS MANANGMENT

It's been said stress is a normal part of life that can either help us learn and grow or can cause us significant problems. Stress releases powerful neurochemicals and hormones that prepare us for action (to fight or flee) and if we don't take action, the stress response can create worse health problems says National Institute of Mental Health (NIMH). And, prolonged, uninterrupted, unexpected, and unmanageable stresses are the most damaging types of stress. There is a lot of evidence showing stress can be manage by seeking support from loved ones, regular exercise, meditation or other relaxation techniques, strutted timeouts, and learning new coping strategies to create predictability in our lives.

Many believes that a increase in times of stress is a maladaptive way of coping with stress, drugs, pain medicines, alcohol, smoking, and eating, actually worsen the stress and can make us more reactive (sensitive) to further stress. While there are promising treatments for stress, the management of stress depends on the ability and willingness of a person to make the changes necessary for a healthy lifestyle.

In addition, stress is simply a fact of nature, forces from the inside or outside world affecting the individual. Most people respond to stress in ways that affect the individual as well as their environment. Because of the overabundance of stress in our modern lives, we usually think of stress as a negative experience, but from a biological point of view, stress can be a neutral negative or positive experience. In general, stress is related to both external and internal factors, says NIMH.

External factors include the physical environment, including your job, your relationships with others, your home, and all the situations, challenges, difficulties, and expectations you're confronted with on a daily basis. On the other hand, internal factors determine your body's ability to respond to, and deal with the external stress. Internal factors influence your ability to handle stress such as your nutritional status, overall health and fitness levels, emotional well-being, and the amount of sleep and rest you get.

Experts believe stress has driven evolutionary change. Therefore, the species that adapted best to the cause of stress (stressors) have survived and evolved into the plant and animal kingdoms we now observe. It's been said that man is the most adaptive creature on the planet because of the evolution of the human brain, especially the part called the neo-cortex. Experts believe this adaptability is largely due to the changes and stressors that we have faced and mastered. In this way, we unlike other animals, can live in any climate or ecosystem, at various altitudes, and avoid the danger of predators.

CLEANING

There is a lot of evidence that shows cleaning can alleviate stress. Cleaning can alleviate stress because it provides relief from clutter. Let's face it, clutter can be stressful, walking into a home that has piles of paper on every surface, stacks of laundry needing to be put away, and random items thrown on the floor feels different than walking into a model home. It's a difference you can feel immediately. While most of us want that neat, ordered home environment, far too many of us live in cluttered surroundings that cause us stress.

According to a pole, less than 10% of the people live in a clutter free home, and over a third lives in surroundings so cluttered that they don't even know where to begin cleaning. Another way cleaning helps prevent stress is when you can find your bill and prevent them from being late. Also, you can avoid replacing items you still have because your kitchen is too cluttered and messy for regular cooking, a little spring cleaning may actually save you money. You may not even realize the ways that a clean house can also be a money saver (which can reduce stress) until you live in one.

In addition, it's been said, when your home is not dirty or messy, you fully appreciate it. I've had many people say that they actually avoid going home because it's a stressful place. Study has shown, inner peace comes more from wanting what you have than from having what you want, unearthing the wonderful haven beneath the dirt and clutter can bring an new level of gratitude for all that you have. To add, the end result of a major cleaning session is a beautiful and clean home, which can be a great stress reliever and the act of cleaning your house can be a stress management technique in itself.

If you incorporate mindfulness into your cleaning, the work can actually be a form of meditation, leaving you more relaxed after you finish. And, if you're one to get into a dancing state as you clean, why not go in the other direction, and turn your cleaning experience into a mini party. As has been mentioned, music has many wonderful stress relief benefits, and playing music as you clean can make the activity much more enjoyable. Play your favorite dance music as you clean, and you may actually work faster and be done sooner.

In all honesty, the act of cleaning, if done right, can bring three added benefit such as getting you a little extra exercise which can be great for relieving stress. When you run up and down the stairs carrying items from room to room, and scrubbing windows and floor can burn calories, release endorphins, and it helps you blow off steam. Spring cleaning is a workout routine that brings many benefits so let have a spring cleaning throughout the year.

"And now that you don't have to be perfect, you can be good."
--John Steinbeck—

TALKING

One of the best remedies for stress can often be as simple as talking. Stress is normally the cause of some sort of problem, whether it is work related, family related etc. We all know what they say about a problem shared, which does have some merit. Altogether, you will find most people add talking in part of their coping techniques when it comes to mental health. It's been said talking a problem through can help you put it in perspective and throw a new, objective view on it. The person who you talk to or confide in can be anyone you think that will be supportive. You might want to speak to a good friend, a partner or a family member. Perhaps you would prefer to speak to a colleague or manager at work.

Or you could even look into talking to your doctor or a trained therapist. It is important to know that however, alone you may feel, there is always someone for you to talk to. If your stress is cause by a person rather than a situation, then there is nothing to stop you from talking it through with the person who is acting as the stressor. This will help you to vent your emotions and feelings, get everything out in to the open rather than bottling it up and it may actually help to clear up some of the problems. The best way to tackle problems that cause you any sort of mental distress is to face them head on, and talking things through with the person who is causing them is an effective way to start tackling this stress. So, whether it is a partner, a family member or a work colleague that is causing you stress it could really help to talk the issues through with them.

In addition, if it is a situation such as bereavement or injury that is causing you to become stressed, then you should consider talking to someone you can confide in and who you think may be able to offer support and advice.

A close friend or family member is always a good choice, also your spouse. However, if you feel that you have nobody to talk to, there are always professionals waiting to help in your area or on the internet that are trained specialist who will be able to talk things through with you. Sharing your burden can often help to lighten the load, and knowing that you have someone to talk things through with and discuss your issues which can often promote a more upbeat and positive feeling. Bottling things up and letting the stress fester is the worst thing that you can do because this fails to solve anything and simply enhances the stress.

Many people are afraid to talk things through because they think that discussing their problems is a sign of weakness. However, it is actually the complete opposite, talking shows that you want to find an effective solutions, and you are prepared to look at all options; and that you are not too proud to ask for help in a time of need.

"I was always fascinated by people who are considered completely normal, because I find them the weirdest of all."
--Johnny Depp--

MASSAGE THERAPY

Americans are looking to massage for much more than just relaxation, "says Mary Beth Braun, President of the American Massage Therapy Association (AMTA). Massage therapy can be effective for a variety of conditions as well as stress. If you can't get to a massage therapist, you can still reap many of the benefits of this age old healing practice with your own hands. Several massage experts was consulted to find these simple, self-message techniques that incorporate the best soothing rubs and pressure point applications that massage has to offer. It is suggested to try them on yourself or someone you love throughout the day to boost your energy and increase concentration.

Also, you can use them at night to relax and get a good night's sleep. You'll find the benefits of massage therapy for stress relief are only the beginning. For example, massage therapy can help to relieve tired eyes. This one is great for tired eyes cause from looking at the computer (which can cause stress) it brings circulation to the area and relieve sinus pressure, eye stain, and headaches, says Dale Grust, President of the New York Chapter of the American Massage Therapy Association and a licensed massage therapist in New Paltz, N.Y., for 23 years.

Here is how it's done. Close your eyes, place your thumbs under your eyebrows, starting at the inside corner of each eye socket. Press and gently move the thumbs in tiny circles, working slowly towards the outside soft your eyebrows and continuing this movement all around your eyes, ending back at the bridge of your nose. Repeat this several times, spending a little extra time at the indentation of the inner eye socket, where the bridge of the nose meets the ridge of the eyebrows an especially tender point on many people says the

AMTA. To add, for relief to ease headaches and tension try Massage Therapy to Ease Headaches and Tension.

    Start by placing your thumbs on your cheekbones close to your ears, and use your fingertips to gently apply pressure and rub the temples (the soft spot between the corner of your eye and your ear). Using very firm pressure and a tiny circular motion, gradually move your fingers up along your hairline until they meet in the middle of your forehead, massaging your entire forehead and scalp as you inch along says the AMTA.

"Some people feel the rain. Others just get wet."
--Bob Marley--

VENTING

One great way that is use to relieve stress is to let it all come flowing out. Anger is one way that can happen, but certainly not the right way. There are other ways to let how you feel flow out that are much better, this is called venting. When someone vents they are letting their stress out. Many people love to vent through writing poetry. Others find that they can vent through painting, drawing, and other forms of the arts. Writing is a very effective way to vent, especially when it is done journal style.

As I suggested earlier, a journal is a way to vent that is safe because you can write anything. When people can write down what they are feeling inside, they allow themselves to get it all out by venting it onto the paper. After they are done many do find that what was once inside of them is now out, and on the paper. Some people take it further and burn or bury the paper. It is said it makes people feel better. Journal (as we will continue to discuss throughout this book) writing can be very beneficial to those who are feeling stress as well as other mental illnesses.

Again, physical activities such as walking, riding a bicycle, engaging in a sport, or even cleaning can also help greatly to reduce stress. When some people are stressed they eat and we don't want to do that because eating can cause another problem such as obesity which can cause you more stress in the long run. So I often clean my house or my car. Also, I take a long, hot shower or bath this can also help to make you feel a lot better when you are stressed.

In addition, experts believe, pain gives us the gift of growth in a hidden package. It's been said that something is shouting out for a change. If we pause and open this gift, a great secret of freedom and love can be revealed.

Sometimes when the pain is large enough, we have no choice but to look at it anyway. My largest pains have helped to open the greatest growths in my life. Hey, it's worth a shot, right: Finding a healthy way to vent can even help to relieve anxiety, something more and more of us are suffering from in these times.

Study has shown, those who don't find a healthy way of venting often stuffs it inside until they explode one day or get into the habit of finding ways to numb themselves, such as eating. Venting can help to truly relieve stress, which is known to cause many ailments and "diseases" in our bodies. Once the energy has been expressed, you can rest in the stillness, while still connected to the power of emotion, to reach the greatest levels of clarity possible.

Experts suggest, this is where our insight is at a natural high. With the power of the openness we have after pain, our greatest growth can happen. We can release the ties to these situations and grow beyond them. Here are some other ways to help vent out frustrations, cry, write, exercise, talk, and create art.

"So often times it happens that we live our lives in chains and we never even know we have the key."

--The Eagles--

BUILD RELATIONSHIPS

The facts show there are many different ways to relieve stress that work, but one sure way to relieve stress is to build relationships. For example, here is how one person spends a Saturday. First they start a Saturday night get together with some people at their church where they picked a house or apartment and spent time eating, playing games and talking with each other. Each time more and more people showed up, and each time they have even more fun that will last. Some would play fun stuff like the crowd favorite called "village" where one person would narrate story and the rest would have to find out who the murderer was. Those nights were fun because they were active, and they were spending quality time with each other and everyone was happy.

In addition, I was told the coolest thing about those nights though were a few weeks after they began those, their friendships grew much deeper than they had. Some noticed soon after that their stress levels were going down and they had a much better outlook on their day to day life. They feel their friends helped bear their burdens by talking and praying with them and they would help bear theirs. For me, I have a friend that have fish fry's every Friday. This is where we play some of the same games, but mostly a lot of card playing. This helps me when I am stressed as well.

A researcher at the Medical University of Vienna spread some good news in honor of National Hug Day (yes, we have a National Hug day it's on January 21 this is not a public holiday). He pointed out that hugging someone you care about can ease stress and anxiety, lower blood pressure and even boost memory. But hugging a stranger can have the opposite effect. While the association between hugging and your health isn't new, it's especially relevant during Valentine's Day with many couples hugging to cuddle away the frigid temperatures sweeping across much of the nation.

    Experts believe it all comes back to the hormone oxytocin. A simple embrace seems to increase levels of the "love hormone," which has been linked to social bonding. The oxytocin boost seems to have a greater calming effect on women than men says USA Today. In one study, the stress-reducing effects of a brief hug in the morning carried throughout a tough work day, USA Today reported.

    Perhaps the best news of all is that hugging isn't the only way getting close to your valentine can boost your health. A few others also have big benefits such as cuddling, call it an extending hug, cuddling also releases stress easing oxytocin, which can reduce blood pressure and bond you with your mate says Huff Post.

"I used to think the worst thing in life was to end up all alone. It's not. The worst thing in life is to end up with people that make you feel alone."
                                           --Robin Williams--

YOGA

Experts believe, dating back over 5000 years, yoga is the oldest defined practice of self development. The methods of classical yoga include ethical disciplines, physical, postures, breathing control and meditation. Traditionally an Eastern practice, it's now becoming popular in the West. In fact, many companies, especially in Britain, are seeing the benefit of yoga, recognizing that relaxed workers are healthier and more creative, and are sponsoring yoga fitness programs. Yoga, which derives its name for the word, "yoke" to bring together does just that bringing together the mind, body and spirit.

But, whether you use yoga for spiritual transformation or for stress management and physical well being, the benefits are numerous and the process is the same. Yoga professionals said the practice of yoga involves stretching the body and forming different poses, while keeping breathing slow and controlled and the body becomes relaxed and energized at the same time. There are various styles of yoga, some moving through the poses more quickly, almost like an aerobic workout, and other styles relaxing deeply into each pose. It is said, some have a more spiritual angle, while others are used purely as a form of exercise.

Additinally, everyone can see physical benefits from yoga, and its practice can also give psychological benefits, such as stress reducing and a sense of well being, and spiritual benefits, such as a feeling of connectedness with God or spirit, or a feeling of transcendence. Certain poses can be done just about anywhere and a yoga program can go for hours or minutes, depending on one's schedule. Yoga does require some commitment of time and is more difficult for people with certain physical limitations. Some people feel self-conscious doing some of the poses.

Also, yoga classes can be expensive, although it is possible, and perhaps more challenging, to learn from a book or video. Some individuals prefer doing yoga at home. I've been told it is easier and private to do yoga in your home if you don't like to be around a group of people. So let's get started reducing stress today.

> *""The guilt I felt for having a mental illness was horrible. I prayed for a broken bone that would heal in six weeks. But that never happened. I was cursed with an illness that nobody could see and nobody knew much about."*
>
> *--Andy Behrman--*

ACUPUNCTURE

According to research, acupuncture is a therapy developed over 5000 years ago in China. It's one of several modalities of treatment practiced under Oriental Medicine (OM) often also referred to as Traditional Chinese Medicine (TCM). The facts show, during treatment, tiny sterile needles are inserted into specific points on the body to adjust the flow of energy, called Qi. According to Oriental Medicine theory, the Qi flows through energy pathways call Meridians. These meridians connect the surface of the body to the internal organs by needling acupuncture points. The function of the internal organs can be adjusted affecting both mental and physical aspects of the patient.

Although some people suggest acupuncture help relieve their stress, scientist believe acupuncture really does reduce stress levels. In the first study of its kind, a team found the ancient Chinese therapy reduces levels of a protein linked to chronic stress. Researchers say it might help explain the sense of well-being many people receive from the therapy and it could offer a proven treatment for stress.

Also, when dealing with the complications of modern life it may require some form of stress management. Experts believe, acupuncture can be an ideal therapy to use in conjunction with lifestyle changes to help you combat stress and enter a more harmonious state. According to Chinese therapy, when your body is subject to constant stress, the Qi of the body becomes congested. This stagnation of the flow of Qi cause a variety of physical and mental symptoms, such as anger, depression, cold limbs, irritable bowel syndrome (IBS), tight tendons and muscles, headaches, and pain.

In a U.S. study, experts tested the effect of acupuncture of blood levels of the protein neuropeptide Y (NPY), which is secreted by sympathetic nervous system in humans. This system is involved in the "flight or fight" response to acute stress, resulting in constriction of blood flow to all parts of the body except to the heart, lungs and brain (organs most needed to react to danger). Chronic stress, however, can cause elevated blood pressure and cardiac disease. She said: "it has long been thought that acupuncture can reduce stress, but this is the first study to show molecular proof of this benefit." "We were surprised to find what looks to be a protective effect against stress". The study is published online in the journal Experimental Biology and Medicine.

"Once you're labeled as mental ill, and that's in your medical notes, then anything you say can be discounted as an artifact of your mental illness."

--Hilary Mantel--

ASK FOR HELP

We know that asking for help is difficult for some people when they are feeling overwhelm with things that have to get done in their life that may cause stress. The following are suggestions to get other family member or close friends involved: Give each person a responsibility, even if it is small, to help spread out the tasks. For example, if taking care of your elderly parents is a responsibility that is overwhelming to you. Call other family members for help. Even if your sister or brother lives 1,000 miles away, make it their responsibility to call your parent once a week to check in or to visit for a week each year to allow you to take your own family vacation.

In addition, speak up, not being able to talk about your needs and concerns creates stress and can make negative feelings worse. Assertive communication (which we talk about in chapter 11) can help you express how you feel in a thoughtful tactful way. Ask for help. People who have a strong network of family and friends manage stress better. Sometimes stress is just too much to handle alone so talking to a friend or family member may help. But you may also want to see a counselor.

Also, if you feel you can't manage stress on your own or you are faced with unbearable stress, remember that there are resources to help. For example, check in with your doctor; experts believe stress can take its toll on your body, increasing your susceptibility to infections and worsening the symptoms of practically any chronic condition. You can always consider counseling as therapy. Stress-management counseling is offered by various types of mental-health professionals. Stress counseling and group-discussion therapy have proven benefits in reduction of stress symptoms and improvement in overall health and attitude. In addition, spend time with those you love.

Countless studies show that people with a balanced, happy social support structure (consisting of friends, family, loved ones, or even pets) experience fewer stress-related symptoms and are better stress managers than people without social support. Your loved ones are also in an excellent position to observe your lifestyle and offer suggestions and help when you need it.

Lastly, take a course, many relaxation programs, mediation techniques, and methods for emotional and physical relaxation are actually learned processes that can be acquires quickly through a class or course with a competent instructor. An added benefit is that you will meet others with similar goals and interests that you can talk to.

"I had some experience in dealing with people who have mental illness and depression, but I didn't see the signs in myself. I couldn't ask for help because I didn't know I needed help."

--*Clara Hughes*--

READ

As I have said, reading is the great way to pass your time and a great way to relax and reduce stress. When you pick up a book and read it, it will take your mind off whatever is causing the stress for a short time. A book can take you to any place you would like to go. Why not go to a South Pacific island with miles of beaches or the top of the Arctic. Maybe try going back in time or into the future as far as you want.

Also, you can read about someone you are interested in, there are biographies and memoirs on just about everyone who was/is famous or important. Fantasy is a good way to help get away from all connections with present time stress. Go to another world, time or visit someone else's imagination. Need to laugh try reading a humorous book. There are some very funny books available on a large range of topics. Reading self-help books (like this one) are also good for reducing stress. These books could help you pinpoint what is causing your stress and give you great coping skills techniques on how to relieve your stress. And, for the non-reader there are books for you also, try reading up on new ideas, how-to-books and technical information on your favorite hobby. For example, say your hobby is gardening, look up and read what new techniques there are available. Read the seed book and plan your next garden project.

In addition, for the photographer check out the latest in cameras or styles of photographs that is currently popular. Start a hobby to help reduce stress by first reading up on where to find it or when and how to do it. What makes reading so good it's a year round activity so when you cannot do your normal stress reducing activity read about it. Reading can also help reduce stress by providing answers to problems.

By reading books it can give advice or instructions on how to solve the problem. When the problem is solved you will feel more relaxed and the stress will melt away. Stress about weight problems can be helped by reading about health, or diet and exercise books. You may find your way to total fitness or back to where you want to be with advice from books.

Also, do you spend too much time eating out because you cannot cook? Here is a good chance to learn to cook from books. When your stress starts to affect your concentration try reading, it will help you to focus and concentrate and exercise you mind. By exercising your mind your ability to concentrate and remembering things will improve. This will also help reduce stress. It's been said reading will also improve your spelling, vocabulary, and writing which will make you feel more confident and reduce stress.

"I know of people who don't believe it, but depression is an illness, but unlike, say, a broken leg, you don't know when it'll get better."

--Marian Keyes--

STRESS BALLS

A stress ball is a small, rubber, gel-filled ball that fits in the palm of the hand. Stress balls come in a wide assortment of shapes and colors and can even be customized, such as being painted with the owner's name. Other stress balls may not be true "balls" but have another shape, such as a heart or a puppy. It is not uncommon for stress balls to be handed out during business meetings, especially in high-intensity corporate environments. Although they may not appear to be effective at first glance, many people use stress balls as a strong stress reliever. To use a stress ball, you first take the stress ball and put it in the palm of your hand. You wrap your fingers around it and simply squeeze that's all to it. You'll notice while you are squeezing that the ball's foamy texture will give, and start molding to the shape of your fingers, this is a process that often feels enjoyable. You squeeze for a few seconds, and then release your fingers from around the ball. It is said with this physical release comes the release of emotional stress and physical tension.

In addition, many people use stress balls for progressive muscle relaxation. Meaning, you squeeze your hand around the stress ball and hold for several seconds, they repeat that process several times, squeezing harder with each repetition. These repetitions induce progressive muscle relaxation because each time you squeeze harder around the ball, the more you relax afterward. Many people do this process while they are at work, especially in the middle of the day when they feel they need a break. Other people use a stress ball right after they come home, to relieve themselves of work-related stress. As it stands, there is no right or wrong way to use a stress ball.

Also, the stress ball relives stress by distracting you; while you are squeezing a stress ball, you can concentrate on what your hands are doing instead of on the source of your tension. It is said it will help to shrink your worry down to a manageable size because it won't be the only thing occupying your mind. Also, stress balls provide a mini workout. Fitness experts believe squeezing the ball is a form of exercise for your arm. It helps to improve your circulation and increases the flow of oxygen to the brain. This can relieve a racing heart rate and help to steady your breathing, which are two common physical symptoms of a heavy amount of stress.

    Lastly, a stress ball can make you happy as well, whether stress balls have novelty shapes or whimsical sayings on them, they can cheer you up, at least for a brief period of time. This mood boost can help to calm you down. They can help you meditate, if you squeeze the ball tightly and then let go, you're actually tightening then relaxing your arm muscle. This can be a good source of meditation if you keep your focus on the movement and squeeze and release for at least 5 minutes.

"Sometimes I say the medication is even tougher than the illness."

--Sanya Richards-Ross--

TAKE A NAP

It's been reported that many people experience a natural increase in drowsiness in the afternoon, about 8 hours after walking. Research shows that you can make yourself more alert, reduce stress, and improve cognitive functioning with a nap. Taking a mid-day sleep, or "power nap" during the day, means more patience, less stress, better reaction time, increased learning, more efficiency, and better health. Here's what you need to know about the benefits of sleep and how a power nap can help you.

Research shows, the body needs 7-8 hours of sleep per day, 6 hours or less triples your risk of a car accident. Interestingly, too much sleep such as more than 9 hours can actually be harmful for your health; recent studies show that those who sleep more than 9 hours per day don't live as long as their 8 hour-sleep counterparts. Many experts advise us to keep the nap between 15 to 330 minutes, because sleeping longer gets you into deeper stages of sleep, from which it's more difficult to awaken. Also, longer naps can make it more difficult to fall asleep at night, especially if your sleep deficit is relatively small.

However, research has shown that a 1 hour nap has many more healing effects than a 30 minute naps and gives you a much greater improvement in cognitive functioning. The key to taking a longer nap is to get a sense of how long your sleep cycle are, and try to awaken at the end of a sleep cycle. (It's actually more the interruption of the sleep cycle that makes you groggy, rather than the deeper states of sleep). Researchers discovered there are pros and cons to each length of sleep, you may want to let your schedule decide. If you only have 15 minutes to spare, take them. But if you could work in an hour nap, you may do well to complete a whole sleep cycle, even if it means less sleep benefit of reducing stress and helping you relax a little, which can give you more energy to complete the tasks of your day. Here are some tips for more effective napping and sleep at night: Avoid caffeine after 3pm because it's a stimulant that can disrupt your sleep and stay in your system longer than you think. If you don't want to nap a long time, set an alarm. If you don't have time for a power nap, or don't feel comfortable napping during the day, try meditation; it gives your body a rest and produces slower brain waves similar to sleep.

"People who attend support groups who have been diagnosed with a life-challenging illness live on average twice as long after diagnosis as people who don't."
--Marianne Williamson--

ARTS AND CRAFT

From the time that man began recording time the creative arts have been used as unique forms or expression, communication and release. Just think of the stick figures found on the cave walls of our earliest ancestors. In the 21st century, researchers discovered how crafts have a healing therapy for people with illnesses for both physical and psychological. It's been said, patients with cancer, for instance, are encouraged to paint as well as taught to visualize their bodies fighting off malignant cells and to pour their thoughts and emotions into journals. Also, abused children are asked to draw pictures to help therapists gain access to their feelings and fears. Arts and crafts are even used as part of the therapeutic rehabilitation of the disabled, the mentally disadvantaged and those with substance abuse problems and to engage the elderly.

Further, the best news is that you don't have to be ill to benefit, "we're now finding that crafts are beneficial for healthy people, too," says Gail McMeekin, MSW, author of the in spring books the 12 secrets of Highly Creative Women and The Power of Positive Choices. "Thanks to their ability to tune you into yourself and your feelings, crafts clearly have physical, psychological and spiritual powers" Adds Diane Erickson, a California fabric artist, teacher and pattern designer, "Crafts are a way of valuing yourself a giving to yourself, they allow you to express what's inside." According to Robert Reiner, PhD, a New York University psychologist and the study's author, the findings prove what crafters already know. Crafts de-stress. "The act of performing a craft is incompatible with worry, anger obsession and anxiety," he says, "crafts make you concentrate and focus on the here and now and distract you from everyday pressures and problems.

They're stress-busters in the same way that meditation, deep breathing, visual imagery and watching fish are."

"Through my illness I learned rejection. I was written off. That was the moment I thought, Okay, game on. No prisoners. Everybody's going down."
--Lance Armstrong--

STRESS RELIEF GAMES

Crossword puzzle book is one of Americans favorite pass time. It's been suggested, to buy a crossword puzzle book for your child because it is the best way to increase their mental ability and relieve stress. For children, first start with an easy level puzzle like I did with my grandchildren and then you can buy difficult ones as they go on solving each stage. They'll surely find it interesting (my grandson did) and you can also help them if they don't know the answer. Computer Games and computers always interest children, or how about a few PC GAMES. They are definitely going to relieve their stress and increase concentration, but remember they might get addicted to these so make sure you indulge them in other activities too along with computer games.

Also, you can down load some good games from the internet and store them to play later. These games will take you away from your routine and therefore away from the tensions. Stress relief games are very much similar to other relaxation techniques like meditation and yoga. While playing these games, you will completely forget the thoughts that burden your mind, thereby affecting your physical and mental health. Here are more stress relief games that you and your friends and family can play. Such as, the facts show, these games help individuals open up in front of others and feel free. The name of this game is called "Lie Detector:" Each one of you must take a piece of paper and write 3-5 things about yourself, one of which must be a lie. When each member of the group has finished writing, the fun part of the game begins. One of you will read aloud the things that they have written about themselves; while the other members have to tell which one is a lie. This is a fun game that will help you to know about each other better and you will also know how much others know about you.

In addition, another game to help release stress is board games. A board game needs a lot of concentration and focus, and they need to be played with a specific strategy. You can opt for the most common board game, i.e., chess or others like monopoly, checkers, scrabble, etc. Through some of these games are easy to play, each game has its rules and you definitely forget other things while trying to win the game. And, another game you can play is called "Who Likes What." This is a game in which you have to decide a category. It can be anything, like movies, actors, songs, games, etc. Now, each one has to write a list consisting of their favorites in this category. For example, if the category is movies, write down ten favorite movies. Once everyone is done, collect all the lists and mix them in a bowl. Now, one of you can be the leader, pick one list and read aloud the items on it. You have to guess whose list this can be. Also, if you are an outdoor person outdoor games can be a good stress releaser if the weather is right. There are a number of outdoor games, like badminton, golf, volley ball, etc., which can be played in groups. Moreover, these games give you good physical exercise while having a fun time with the group members. I hope I gave you some good game ideas that will help you relieve some stress.

"I think that that's the wisest thing-to prevent illness before we try to cure something."

--Maya Angelou--

PRIORITIZE

Prioritization is the essential skill that you need to make the very best use of your own efforts. It is said when you prioritize it can help to illuminate stress. It's also a skill that you need to create calmness and space in your life so that you can focus your energy and attention on the things that really matter. It's particularly important when time is limited and demands are seemingly unlimited.

Also, It helps you to allocate your time where it's most needed and most wisely spent, freeing you up from less important task that can be attended to later or quietly dropped. With good prioritized skills (and careful management of reprioritized tasks) you can bring order to chaos, massively reduce stress, and move towards a successful conclusion. Without it, you'll flounder around drowning in competing demands. It is said, prioritization based on project value or profitability is probably the most commonly used and rational basis for prioritization. Whether this is based on subjective guess at value or a sophisticated financial evaluation, it often gives the most efficient results.

Moreover, prioritizing introduces two of the most important techniques of stress management; taking a step back and doing one thing at a time. It doesn't just help people manage a heavy workload, prioritizing can also break some of its most vicious circles.

In addition, the act of prioritizing forces someone to think about items individually again. Considering tasks separately brings them back down to size. It dispels the power and magic they had as part of an intimidating whole. Once the stressful mass is broken up, individual task can be laid end-to-end in an orderly row so they can be picked off one by one.

This brings in that second component of stress management doing one thing at a time. Like viewing tasks individually, focusing on one thing reverses some of the unhelpful patterns stress creates. When people are stressed, time makes it hard to keep your mind from jumping to whatever isn't getting done at the time. The result is that few tasks have your full concentration. A lack of concentration risks missing vital information or making mistakes which need even more time to remedy. Taking small steps in multiple directions robs you of the sense of progress that comes from wiping something off the list.

And, prioritize those things that cannot be eliminated. Do only what is absolutely necessary and no more. During recovery and de-stressing times, get the most important to do list and if it's not in the top three, then they probably aren't that critical and it won't be earth shattering if they have to wait until a day or two later. Research has shown prioritizing is a good habit to get into even when the work isn't stressful. It has a preventative effect which keeps unnecessary clutter getting through in the first place. It also serves as a type of review or stock-taking which can refresh your view of the work you do and what's important to you.

"I enjoy convalescence. It is the part that makes the illness worthwhile."

--George Bernard Shaw--

PRAY/CHURCH

As was previously stated, prayer at home or at church is effective in reducing stress as well. Here is an example of a prayer to relieve stress. You can personalize it for you and your God or say it for all that is in need. "Father of Love, hear my prayers for the sick members of our community and for all who are in need. Amid mental suffering, stress and anxiety may they find consolation in your healing presence and show your mercy and free son cast sprits; may these people find peace and lasting health, we ask this through the (your God name) Lord Jesus who healed those who believed Amen. In Dr. Lee new book, The Super Stress Solution, Dr Roberta Lee devotes a section to the topic of spirituality and prayer. "Research shows that people who are more religious or spiritual use their spirituality to cope with life," notes Dr. Lee. "They're better able to cope with stress, they heal faster from illness, and they experience increased benefits to their health and well-being.

Also, on an intellectual level Spirituality connects you to the world, which in turn enables you to stop trying to control things all by yourself. When you feel part of a great whole, it's easy to understand that you aren't responsible of everything that happens in life." And among the research she cites is one study of approximately 126,000 people that found that the people who frequently attended services increased their odds of living by 29 percent. Another study conducted by the National Institute of health Care Research (NIHR) illustrated that the Canadian college students who were connected to their campus ministries visited doctors less often and were less stress during difficult times than the other students.

The students who had strong religious correlations also had higher positive feelings, lower levels of depression, and were better equipped at handling stress.

"Mental illness, of course, is not literally a 'thing'-or physical object-and hence it can 'exist' only in the same sort of way in which other theoretical concepts exist."
--Thomas Szasz--

WALKING TO RELIEVE STRESS

As has been mentioned, exercise is a proven stress-manage technique because it helps to take your mind off of stressful life situations. It also assists in protecting the heart from the harmful effects of stress. The one exercise that is said to help when you are stress is walking. The power of walking as a stress-reliever and mood enhancer is often underestimated. Walking is such a simple exercise, one that most people do without thinking.

However, walking as a conscious form of exercise has been known to reduce stress and depression. Walking briskly is one form of exercise that has been known to relieve stress. A short, brisk walk can do wonders for shifting your attention away from a day's challenges and toward appreciating the present moment. While walking, you may notice beautiful scenery, a friendly dog or a mom with her cute babies. These experiences and others may help you to appreciate the good things in life and connect you with others. Often, if you are feeling down or under a great deal of stress and feel lost in your own mind, connecting with others is soothing and a good reminder to see the bigger picture.

In addition, even if the walk is done in solitude and without interacting with others, just being in nature and moving the body can have a positive effect on the body and the mind. Stress management studies show that if you make a plan and carry it to completion, this helps you to feel more in control and gives you a sense of accomplishment. As it applies to walking, it is said if you are new to exercise, you might consider walking just ten minutes per day to start out. If doing this every day seems difficult, you might limit it to a few days a week.

Soon you might find that you are enjoying yourself and wanting to increase your walk by a few minutes each time or more days per week. The day is to start with a manageable activity and accomplish each small goal, then build on its. Here are some ways to enjoy your walk; you can select a path that is free of noise and pollution. Walking in scenic locations helps to uplift the mood. Also, you can listen to your favorite music while walking this has been known to reduce stress as well.

In one study that observed students who listened to a gentle piece of music while performing a stressful task, music was found to lower the heart rate and blood pressure, and decrease feelings of anxiety. Therefore, combining walking, beautiful scenery and soothing music is a helpful strategy for reducing stress.

"The number one root of all illness, as we know, is stress."
--Marianne Williamson--

Chapter 6

ANGER MANAGEMENT

Do you have a short fuse or find yourself getting into frequent arguments and fights? Anger is a normal, healthy emotion, but when chronic, explosive anger spirals out of control, it can have serious consequences for your relationships, your health, and your state of mind.

According to West Virginia University, The Student Center for Health in Anger Management Techniques, when you gain insight about the real reasons for your anger and learn these anger management tools, you will learn to keep your temper from hijacking your life. The emotion of anger is neither, good or bad. It's perfectly healthy and normal to feel angry when you've been mistreated or wronged. The feeling isn't the problem; it's what you do with it that makes a difference. Anger becomes a problem when it harms you or others. If you have a hot temper, you may feel like it's out of your hands and there's little you can do to tame the beast.

The good news is, you have more control over your anger than you think. You can learn to express your emotions without hurting others, and when you do, you'll not only feel better, you'll also be more likely to get your needs met. Moreover, mastering the art of anger management takes work, but just like anything else, the more you practice, the easier it will get and the payoff can be huge. When you learn to control your anger and express it appropriately it can help you build better relationships, achieve your goals, and lead a healthier, more satisfying life.

Also, if your anger seems to be spiraling out of control, remove yourself from the situation for a few minute or for as long as it takes you to cool down. A brisk walk, a trip to the gym, or a few minutes listening to some music should allow you to calm down to release pent up emotion, and then approach the situation with a cooler head. Consider professional help if you feel constantly frustrated and angry no matter what you try. Get help if your temper causes problems at work or in your relationships. Try to avoid new people if you feel like you can't control your temper so you will not get in trouble with the law due to your anger, and you can avoid getting led to physical violence. Anger is a very powerful emotion that can stem from feelings of frustration, hurt, annoyance, or disappointment.

Lastly, it is a normal human emotion that can range from slight irritation to strong rage. Experts believe, suppressed anger can be an underlying cause of anxiety and depression. Anger that is not appropriately expressed can disrupt relationships, affect thinking and behavior patterns, and create a variety of physical problems. Research shows, chronic anger can be linked to problems such as crime, emotional and physical abuse, and other violent behavior.

TOOLS FOR ANGER MANAGEMENT

Work-Out by Jim Messina, Ph.D. contains a variety of strategies for working out the different faces of anger. It is important to use all of these tools during your recovery process as well as recognize the course of the anger cycle so you can use the ANGERS workout system to escape this cycle.

According to Messina, the typical unhealthy anger cycle is: When you express anger in your old "sick" way, the automatic natural response is guilt for hurting the feelings of the person so you immediately feel remorse. You then convince yourself to believe the anger.

However, you still feel resentment over the real or perceived motivation which promoted your anger. If you are again irritated by this or similar motivation, you will express anger again. It is not useful when you are trying to recover from anger to express your anger directly on people in the old sick way which keeps you trapped in the anger cycle. For this reason, Messina suggests using the ANGER workout system when you get angry.

A=ACCEPT
N=NAME
G=GET IT OUT
E=ENERGIZE
R=RESUME

First, it is said you need to accept what you are feeling is anger. There is evidence showing most people often have a tendency to deny these powerful emotions because of their experience with anger in the past has been painful, hurtful, or disastrous, so don't deny your anger. Second, face it head on for what it is says Messina.

Also, you need to name and identify what is getting you so angry. You need to name what it is about the situation that motivates you and is triggering your response. Utilize the ANGER systems to help you to analyze and think out what is going on to get your anger motivated and provoke your anger. Third, you now need to get out of you system by expressive emotional release of anger workout. Get yourself in a private place (if you can) to use one of the following activities to aggressively ventilate your anger on lifeless objects rather than on people.

Yelling in your head silently
Yelling in a car with windows close
Yelling in a room away from others
Yelling into a paper bag or pillow
Beating on pillows, cushions, or mattress'
Hitting a punching bag, weight bag
Screaming in a vacant field or lot
Screaming with a towel in your mouth
Ripping a telephone book, newspaper, or catalog

Forth, once you have aggressively ventilated and experienced emotional release of the anger, you will energize yourself to feel calmer; more relaxed, less anxious, less tense, or less stressed. Aggressive anger work will enable you to be more rational and realistic and better able to use the ANGER systems to promote your recovery says Messina.

Fifth, once you are energized, resume your involvement with the person who motivated your anger and assertively confront the person with how you feel in a calm, cool, rational manner.

"The control center of your life is your attitude."
--Norman Cousins--

ANGER SUPPORT HOTLINE

Anger management hotlines offer support, information, and crisis intervention to anyone involved in an anger-related situation. They may also provide long-tem counseling and referrals to outside agencies for continued services. Experts believe uncontrolled anger is a serious problem that can lead to domestic violence, child abuse, personal injury, pervert damage, criminal activity, and loss of employment.

According to the American institute on Domestic Violence, more than 5 million women are abused every year, and anger and violence account for nearly one-quarter of all middle-class divorces in the United States. It's been said chronic anger can significantly affect health and lead to the development of heart disease, diabetes, depression, and immune system dysfunction. Calling an anger support hotline can help you prevent or escape a potentially dangerous situation and speaking with an anger counselor can help you develop the coping skills need to control your anger and prevent its harmful effects. People on the other end of the line are trained professionals or caring volunteers with experience resolving conflict and keeping calm under crisis conditions. They are available to help before anger gets out of control and during and anger related crisis. All hotlines are beneficial to those with anger management problems and can provide support and information when anger gets out on control and during anger related crisis. Hotlines are beneficial to those with anger management problems and to their loved ones as well.

In addition, anger management support hotlines offer a different perspective on whatever situation making you angry. This can provide you with the opportunity to find a healthy solution to your problem.

Counselors can offer tips on coping with anger and stress to make it less likely that you will lose control in the future. Calling a support hotline allows you to talk over your problems and vent your anger, which is often enough to diffuse a potentially dangerous situation. Speaking with a professional can help you control your anger and prevent it from escalating to a dangerous level.

Also, anger management counselors receive training in relaxation techniques and crisis intervention.
Counselors can offer you a safe outlet for your anger, talk you down from a potentially dangerous emotional cliff, or contact family members to assist you. Anger management counselors are able to contact the authorities on your behalf if you feel you are a danger to yourself or others, and they will remain on the line with you until help arrives.

"The problem with the stigma around mental health is really about the stories that we tell ourselves as a society. What is normal? That's just a story that we tell ourselves."
--Matthew Quick--

MUSIC THERAPY

As I have said, music can be a helpful tool in learning to manage strong emotions. Music therapy is far from the first thing we associate with anger management. However, music's expression of emotions through the stories we hear in songs can help to raise emotional awareness and the awareness of options for expressing them. Research shows, emotional awareness is the first part of any anger management training program, whether the program is tailored to individuals or groups. In order to manage anger a person needs to know just how angry or upset they are.

For example, it's been said, songs that portray stories can be used to "diagnose" how angry the person in the song seems to be and talking about the situation in a song can give you a bit of detachment from the emotion that they may feel when they themselves are in such a situation. After focusing on the song, you can personalize the situation to describe the feelings he/she might experience in situation. It is in this capacity that anger management and music therapy are so incredibly effective. Songs also can be used to pick out the emotions contributing to anger.

In addition, professionals believe, anger is often emotions of grief, sense of loses or injustice, or perhaps jealousy or shame that can be identified in a song or in the client when in a similar situation. Sometimes a music therapist may ask a client to choose a song that mirror a situation in the client's life. This helps the therapist and the client to explore the emotions behind the anger. The same examining of stories in songs helps to identify the thoughts behind emotions, and which thoughts can contribute to escalation in the clients. These thoughts, which are sometimes irrational, can then be worked on and sometimes changed.

Again, this is another reason why anger management and music therapy are so effective when combined. In your early anger management and music therapy it is to help you be able to rate your stress level. You and the therapist work on a scale that ranges from 1 to 10 and this allows them to become aware of your baseline level. This also helps you to know when you need to engage in preventative de-stressing techniques like exercise, meditation, or recreational pursuits.

In addition, this anger management technique also helps you to recognize when you are escalating and need to take an immediate "time out" away from the source of stress. Also, songs can be used to describe the situations that you have the most difficulty with in keeping your cool. So you see there are many ways anger management and music therapy can work together to raise awareness of feelings, to depicting emotions felt in different situations, or to describe many options for expression of emotions, as well as presenting techniques for venting and calming.

"A winner is one who accepts his failures and mistakes, picks up the pieces, and continues striving to reach his goals."
--Dexter Yagar--

UNDERSTANDING/COMPASSION

Obviously, becoming physically aggressive in harmful ways is a bad strategy, one that could lead to serious consequences for you and other people. But what about the more harmless form of venting, like punching a pillow? Research suggests that letting off steam, even in the most harmless forms, is not an effective way to control your anger all the time. In fact, these supposedly harmless forms of venting have been shown to increase aggressive behavior later on. So while you may temporarily feel better, be careful because the act of venting can lead you to have more difficulty with your anger down the road.

In the past, therapists have advised people to do things like go punch a pillow, but we now know that this isn't always the best advice. So it doesn't help to suppress anger, and venting it only leads to increasing your arousal, so, what's a person to do? Experts believe, there are two options, and both seem to work well. One, mentally, we must very quickly evaluate the situation. When you wait too long, the arousing chemicals kick in and it's much harder. We can short circuit our rage by challenging our interpretation of events, aiming to reduce our perceived threat. Our job is to find some understanding, even compassion in the situation. This works up to medium levels of anger. Research shows, at high level, we may be "cognitively incapacitated" and reframing our thoughts won't work. Then we need physical action to cool down. We have to wait out the adrenaline surge in a setting where there aren't likely to be further triggers. Such as, going for a long walk or exercising.

Also, using techniques such as abdominal breathing, and muscle relaxation (techniques are located in this book) works just by changing your physiology. But a cooling down period won't work if we keep thinking angry thoughts.

We have to distract ourselves with TV, music, and reading is said to work, but indulgences such as shopping or eating don't have much effect and alcohol escalates anger into violence. So don't automatically "let it out". Stop to evaluate your thoughts, take a breather, and let your chemicals calm down. You'll have a much better chance of successful handling the situation. Express it (the right way).

Sometimes we get angry because the same things keep happening over and over, such as our partner interrupts us, a friend stands us up or a co-worker keeps making mistakes. Addressing these problems in a moment of anger can make things worse. But it is important to bring it up in the right way because the other person involved may not realize they are making you angry or may be able to change things to improve the situation.

"Don't' let life discourage you; everyone who got where he is had to begin where he was."

--Richard L. Evans--

REMOVE YOURSELF

Take a deep breath and remove yourself from the situation. If it's about to blow, on someone's presence, verbally or physically, remove yourself. Walk away, excuse yourself. Clear your head over it, before you are about to blow. Think about the situation and try to make total sense of what, or why you are so mad. Chances are you're overreacting and blowing the situation out of control. Let your thoughts simmer and make peace of what is making you so angry. The anger is hurting you more than the person. You have to understand this part, sometimes people don't always do something you want so in your mind you try to get even with them and take it out on them. Even if you try to get back at them, it's going to still take more out of you, not them. So they win again. The easy solution is to compromise and be the winner.

To add, stressful events don't excuse anger, but understanding how these events affect you can help you take control of your environment and avoid unnecessary aggravation. Look at your regular routine and try to identify activities, times of day, people, places, or situations that trigger irritable or anger feelings. For example, maybe you get into a fight every time you go out for drinks with a certain group of friends.

Or maybe the traffic on your daily commute drives you crazy. Then think about ways to avoid these triggers or view the situation differently so it doesn't make your blood boil and step away. Words said in anger are rarely well thoughts out and you can't take it back. If you find yourself really angry at a partner or co-worker, sometimes its better just to admit those feelings and walk away to think about your response. It's fine to say, "I just need a few minutes to be alone and get my thoughts together". Think about it; from my experience, sometimes logic is anger's worst enemy.

We're often angry about things that we've misinterpreted or blown out of proportion. We may think a friend did something on purpose to upset us, but when we look closer at the situation we realize it was unintentional. Or something that really outraged us, like a roommate eating the last of your favorite snack, may seem less important when you think about it.

"The strongest predictor of unhappiness is anyone who has had a mental illness in the last 10 years. It is an even stronger predictor of unhappiness than poverty-which also ranks highly."

--Polly Toynbee--

TRIGGERS AND DISTRACTION

It's been noted, triggers are very important when it comes to emotions. So let's talk about triggers as it relates to anger. You may never be able to completely get rid of, avoid or change the people and things that make you angry. But you can learn to recognize your anger "triggers" and develop healthier ways to deal with how anger makes you feel and act. That's what anger management is about.

Researchers discovered some anger management strategies that can help you keep your anger triggers from tipping you over the edge. Distraction is an effective anger management technique because it helps keep your mind off the thing that made you angry.

Here are 10 distracting activities you can try.

One, play a board game, work on a puzzle, paint, draw or sculpt, play with your pet, call/text/chat with a friend, play a computer game, read a book, watch a movie, cook, and meditate. It is said, to be effective, a good distraction should fully engage you mind. For example, TV may not be distracting enough to fully get your mind off what made you angry in the first place. How about counting to 10? Counting to 10 is not very distracting because you probably can do it in you sleep, it's very automatic. Instead, try counting backwards from 100 by 7's. Some people even say the alphabets backwards. Some people punch a pillow, or a wall. I don't think that's a good idea because of the fact that you might break your hand; do you really want to train your brain to hit something when you get angry? More importantly, what happens when there is no pillow? Surely you can think of something else.

In addition, just as the name implies, distraction is anything you do to temporarily take your attention off of a strong emotions. Sometimes, focusing on a strong emotion can make it feel even stronger and more out of control. Therefore, by temporarily distracting yourself, you may give the emotion some time to decrease in intensity, making it easier to manage. A key part of the above definition of distraction is the word, temporarily. Distraction is not about trying to escape or avoid a feeling. With distraction, it is implied that you eventually will return to the feeling you were having.

Then, once the intensity of the feeling has reduced, you will try to use another skill to manage the emotion, such as expressive writing (demonstrated in this book). Distraction can keep you safe in the moment by preventing unhealthy behaviors (such as drug use or deliberate self-harm) that occur in response to a strong feeling, as well as making a feeling easier to cope with in the long-run.

"Occupying my mind with complex problems has been my best and most powerful and most reliable defense against my mental illness."

--Elyn Saks--

EMOTIONAL CONTROL

First, just remember nothing makes you mad, people and situations don't make you mad, you choose it. You might not be conscious of it, but in your emotional state you choose it. Just remember, we are a product of our choices, then ask yourself the question, "If something or someone is making you mad, how long do you have to be mad" until they make me un-mad; of course not, you're the one in control. Things like this are exactly what emotional intelligence is about. Second, control what you can, and choose your response based on values. For example, sooner or later, one way or another, this "will" be resolved. When it's over and you look back on your behavior during this difficult time, how would you like to have presented yourself, perhaps with grace and strength?

Or as the example of an intelligent leader who shows others how to behave when the going gets tough. Maybe as someone who behaves even when no one else is watching? Then, behave according to your values. When all is lost always go back to your values and you can never go wrong they will never let you down.

Moreover, self-awareness is an ability to notice what you're feeling and thinking, and why. Little kids aren't very aware of what they are feeling; they just act it out in their behavior. That's why you see them having tantrums when they're mad. But teens and adults have the mental ability to be self-aware. When you get angry, take a moment to notice what you're feeling and thinking.

In addition, self-control is all about thinking before you act. It puts some precious seconds or minutes between feeling a strong emotion and taking an action you'll regret.

Together, self-awareness and self-control allow you to have more choice about how to act when you're feeling an intense emotion like anger. Despite the popular idea that we need to "express" our anger so that it doesn't eat away at us, there's nothing constructive about expressing anger to another person.

Research shows that expressing anger while we are angry actually makes us angrier. This in turn makes the other person hurt, afraid, or angry, and cause a rift in the relationship. So discharge your anger physically if you need to, but then calm yourself and consider what the "message" of the anger before you speak with the other person. When we rehash the situation in our mind it always proves to us that we are right and the other person is wrong, which again makes us angrier as we stew. What works is to find a constructive way to address whatever is making us angry so that the situation is resolved.

"I don't believe you have to have eating disorders and mental illness to screw up."

--Kirstie Alley--

BREATHING TECHNIQUES

Experts believe, the best time to use breathing techniques to manage your angry outbursts is while you are calm and happy. If you can get in the practice of doing this simple, yet effective breathing exercise several times a day while you are calm and in a good mood the positive effect it will have on your emotional balance will speed up quickly. The idea of "nipping your anger in the bud" gives your mind a practiced place or habit to return to when you find yourself out of control. I found that by doing this exercise in the morning, whenever I could during the workday and as I fell asleep made a huge difference in my ability to return to a calmer state of being when I feel my anger creeping up inside.

It's been suggested to do this exercise when you see the first signs of anger building up in you, you'll be able to go to that calm place within yourself quicker than if you don't use this technique.

To start, here's the exercise. According to fitness experts, this is a classic exercise for breathing techniques in a 4 counts, hold for 4 counts and release for 4 counts. Just follow your natural rhythm. Don't force yourself to breathe faster or slower, let it come naturally. Then, close your eyes and imagine the number you are saying in your mind's eye as you're counting. This helps to give you something to focus on until you find the calming effect of the exercise. At first you'll be counting quickly, but don't worry, that is to be expected. Simply continue to do this for several minutes, reminding yourself that with each full cycle of 4-4-4 you are getting closer to that calmer natural state that is inherently yours.

Also, it is suggested to repeat statements such as "I'm getting calmer with each breath cycle" "The more I practiced, the calmer I see myself in the future."

"This is really working I feel so calm." For increased benefit, write down how good you feel in your journal, extending the feeling of peacefulness even longer. Remember that it takes time to change a habit and that your best path to a happier, more relaxed life is to take it one step and one action at a time.

Every day you do this exercise, you'll be one day closer to an improve you. So let's get started on our 4 counts.

"Early diagnosis is so important because the earlier a mental illness can be detected, diagnosed and treatment can begin, the better off that person can be for the rest of his or her life."
--Rosalynn Carter--

LAUGH

It is said you can use laughter to reduce your vulnerability to anger. Most comedians feel laughter is (literally) a painkiller. It can kill both physical and emotional pain, reducing the likely hood that certain situations will make you angry.

Studies compensating some type of neural distraction, relaxation, and laughter found laughter to be most effective in raising a person's pain threshold as well. So bottom line, laughter reduces pain sensitivity and the same is true for anger sensitivity, how touchy you are and how easily you can be provoked to anger. In other words, you're less likely to be annoyed by something if you're in good humor than if you are not. Think of humor as a shield that protects you from the stinging impact of someone else's bad behavior. Some people (like me) seem to have been born with a keen sense of humor. They don't have to try to be funny or make themselves and other people laugh, it just comes naturally. Other people have to look outside themselves to find something to make them laugh.

To add, here are some ways to try that will bring some laughter into your life. If you have a friend with a good sense of humor, spend time with that person as often as you can. Avoid the serious stuff on TV especially the news and watch things that are lighthearted, even to the point of being silly. Find some movies that make you laugh and watch them repeatedly, think of it as therapy. Eat out in places where people tend to be loud, raucous, and having fun. Spend time with pets because they can do the funniest things especially when you get to know them, they can be a riot. Go to a bookstore and buy joke book or watch late night TV. I know it sound silly and stupid but this is just what the doctor ordered at the end of a long stressful day.

Involve yourself in activities that provide good natured fellowship. Keep visual reminders in your home and office of fun times and friends and family. You can also, close your eyes and revisit a situation where you laughed until your sides burst that always works.

"People are always selling the idea that people with mental illness are suffering. I think madness can be an escape. If things are not so good, you maybe want to imagine something better."

--John Forbes Nash, Jr.--

JOURNALING AND ANGER

Journaling has been mentioned for other mental illnesses. But for each mental illness there are pacific ways to journal. Writing about anger is one of the most effective ways to understand, express, learn from, and take positive action in guiding your anger. Through writing, you process the reasons for your anger. Once you know why you're angry, you have more control: you can examine your responses and choose different ones. Also, you can learn from your anger and take positive action to protect yourself from further disappointment or harm. Anger, is in my experience, becomes an emotion that wakes you up and makes you pay attention to yourself. It's difficult to write when you're in immediate danger so I advise waiting until you can sit still.

Then, while you're still feeling the anger, bring it to the page. Here are a few writing prompts to help you get started. Express your anger by putting on papers every negative thoughts, wish and destructive impulse. For example, write about wishing your ex would jump off a cliff or get into a car accident; write out those murder fantasies; doodle all the names you'd like to call that co-worker or situation. You can even slash the pencil across the page, its okay. No one will see what you write, and you can always shred it when you're done. Write until you feel the anger seeping out through your fingers onto the page. Until you're exhausted or, better yet, you can laugh at yourself, just a little. Think about what you are angry about. What happened to hurry you? Was it an act by someone else or a situation out of your control?

Also, free write for ten minutes, beginning with, "I'm angry because.
What does your anger tell you about your life? What does it tell you about yourself? Write a conversation with your anger.

Ask it why it exists and what positive action it wants you to take to feel better. Write several concrete steps you can take along with how you will accomplish them. You can write how you can respond differently or what do you need to do to protect yourself from being hurt again.

For example, if after writing, you decide your response was due to something that happened long ago, in other words, the recent behavior or event didn't actually cause, but triggered your anger you may decide to spend several sessions writing about the original event, or you may decide to seek therapy. If you decide that you need to remove yourself from a harmful situation, write down the actions you need to take.

You can also, free write for ten minutes about all the ways that your anger empowers you to change your life. Beginning with, "My anger empowers me to… Remember, anger can be a negative, destructive emotion, but it does not need to be. When you use writing to process and learn about your anger, you'll have the power to choose what you want to do with it. What do you do with yours?

"Some seek the comfort of their therapist's office, other head to the corner pub and dive into a pint, but I chose running as my therapy."

--Dean Karnazes--

REACTION VS RESPONSE

Experts believe, anger management is being aware of your reactions versus response and reaction is an immediate, almost instinctive approach to a situation we are involved with, or a perception we have. It's something that is done without thinking, something done on impulse, without consideration of what the consequences might be. Here's an example. Let's say you go to a crowded place (a concert, sporting event, bar, nightclub, etc) as you are walking along, you bump into someone. That person looks at you, and before you can say anything, they push you. Why would they do this? They might have the perception that you bumped into them on purpose and that you wanted to start some sort of confrontation. They don't even give you a chance to apologize, or to consider that you bumped into them because you were pushed from behind. They reacted. They pushed you without pausing to think why it happened. It was automatic and thoughtless. It was a reaction.

Now, imagine if the other person paused before pushing you. If they had actually paused, they would have heard your apology and likely would have responded peacefully instead of reacting angrily. When we pause and think about our options, we are responding. Pausing reduces anger: This is what you want to do when you feel angry you want to pause, even if just for a couple of seconds, before you say or do anything. When we pause, we are allowing ourselves to respond appropriately to a situation, rather than reacting and doing something that we might regret later. This is one of the fundamental anger management strategies.

That is, to learn how to pause and take a few seconds, or a few minutes, or even a few hours before dealing with the situation that is triggering your anger. It is said this will also help you gain a deeper insight into your emotions, and may be more effective when trying to manage your anger.

However, reacting is not always the wrong decision. It is not always bad to react because there are situations where there is no time, and you will have to react. This is why you train yourself. You always want to attempt to assess the situation, but if a rock is falling from the sky, you better react and move. Responding is not an excuse to not make a decision. In fact, it is the opposite. Learning how to respond should allow you to make faster decisions and even react better when you need to. You have to understand a situation, and if you start reacting less, your life will get better, because you are now only reacting to things you really need to. You are responding to the rest.

"It is as if my life was magically run by two electric currents; joyous positive and despairing negative—whichever is running at the moment dominates my life, floods it."
                                                                                    --Sylvia Plath--

ASSERTIVE

Being assertive is a core communication skill but with mental illness can sometimes be hard to do. According to communication experts, being assertive means that you express yourself effectively and stand up for your point of view, while also respecting the rights and beliefs others. Being assertive can help boost your self-esteem and earn others respect. This can help with stress management, especially if you tend to take on too many responsibilities because you have a hard time saying no to people. Some people seem to be naturally assertive, but if you're not one of them, you can learn to be more assertive. Because assertiveness is based on mutual respect, it's an effective and diplomatic communication style. Being assertive also shows that you respect yourself because you're willing to stand up for your interests and express your thoughts and feelings. It can demonstrate that you're aware of the rights of others and are willing to work on resolving conflicts.

Of course, it's not just what you say in your message but also how you say it that's important. Assertive communication is direct and respectful. Being assertive gives you the best chance of successfully delivering your message. If you communicate in a way that's too passive or too aggressive, your message may get lost because people are too busy reacting to your delivery.

On the other hand, if your style is aggressive, you may come across as a bully who disregards the needs, feelings and opinions of others. Your may appear self-righteous or superior. Very aggressive people humiliate and intimidate others and may even be physically threatening. You may think that being aggressive gets you what you want but it comes at a cost because it under cuts trusts and mutual respect.

It may result to others resenting you, and leading them to avoid or oppose you. Being assertive is usually viewed as a healthier communication style and offers many benefits. It helps you keep people from walking all over you.

On the flip side, it can also help you from stream rolling others. Behaving assertively can help you to gain self-confidence and self-esteem, understand and recognize your feelings, earn respect from others, improve communication, create win-win situations, improve your decision-making skills, create relationships, and gain more job satisfaction. Learning to be more assertive can also help you effectively express your feelings when communicating with others seems impossible.

"This feeling will pass. The fear is real but the danger is not."
--Cammie McGovern--

EXPECTATIONS

It's been said the way you look at how life affects your response to a situation. Five different people might have five different reactions to the same irritating event. Some people might think that a person acting out at them with road rage is funny, while others might take it as a personal slight, or for others it might be the last straw proving that everyone is out to ruin their day.

In other words, some people have the natural ability to let aggravations role off their back while others get furious when expectations don't go as planned. The problem is that you wish that you could have accomplished things one-way (in this case it's getting to work without any stress), and can't get over what actually occurred. When the expectation isn't met, some people can't get past the moment and shift their aggression towards another person. We all have our expectations of how things should work. We know hopeful and positive expectations can lead to a more optimistic outlook.

However, when we set our expectations of ourselves, or circumstances too high, we can end up constantly feeling frustrated, hurt and angry. Many people think that if they could just get the other person to change his ways, they'd be much happier. Also, anger management experts feel the key aspect to managing your anger is learning how to manage your own expectations to a more realistic level. So how can you adjust your expectations without feeling like you've given up? It's important to realize that not everyone thinks like you. If you start every day expecting that everyone is going to fall in line behind you and accept all your thoughts and ideas, you set yourself up for failure. The successful management of expectations requires that you don't just assume others should know you by now or "understand you", but that you constantly communicate respectfully, calmly and clearly what you need and why because just expecting that your stay at home spouse will have dinner ready when you get home from work, or that your employees will do a project the way you can will create confusion and frustration.

So, instead of flying off the handle, slow down and try to understand the other person's point of view. Listen to them closely and repeat back what you are hearing to make sure it's clear. Having an open and honest discussion can help both sides to feel like their opinion matters and contribute to successful resolution.

"What does your anxiety do? It does not empty tomorrow of its sorrow; but empties today of its strength. It does not make you escape the evil; it makes you unfit to cope with it if it comes."
--Joanne Greenberg--

DON'T STUFF ANGER

The facts show, one standard approach to deal with anger is to hide it. This approach is endorsed by most societies. This approach can prompt people to stuff their anger deep inside and repress it. But there is some evidence that this is a costly strategy. Several studies have shown that stuffing anger inside can have a negative health consequence, such as increasing the risk of heart disease.

On the other hand, it's been said if people try to hide their anger, some anger might be diminished. A second approach to deal with anger is to express it. This view treats anger as a kind of inner pressure or corrosive substance that builds up over time inside the person and does harm unless it is released. Catharsis theory fits in this second approach because it holds that expressing anger produced a healthy release of emotion and is therefore good for the psyche. Unfortunately, scientific evidence shows that venting one's anger only makes things worse. Venting harms the self and others if not done properly. Expressing anger is also linked to higher risk of heart disease, just like stiffing it inside.

However, expressing anger has another drawback, it increase aggression against others, even among people who believe in the value of venting and catharsis, and even when people enjoy their venting and feel some satisfaction from it, aggression becomes more likely after venting innocent by standers.

To add, a positive way of venting is intense physical exercise. When angry, some people go running or try some other form of physical exercise such as kickboxing. Physical exercise is not good for reducing anger but it can help release anger and avoid stuffing it inside.

Experts believe the reason physical exercise doesn't work is that it increases rather than decreases physiological arousal, such as heart rate and blood pressure. When people become angry, they physiological arousal increases, however, that prolonged exercise will eventually reduce anger, if it continues until the person is extremely tired because then the arousal is finally dispersed and people feel too exhausted to feel anger.

"Our society tends to regard as a sickness any mode of thought or behavior that is inconvenient for the system and this is plausible because when an individual doesn't fit into the system it cause pain to the individual as well as problems for the system. Thus the manipulation of an individual to adjust him to the system is seen as a cure for a sickness and therefore as good."

--Theordore Kaczynski--

DON'T ATTACK OR BLAME OTHERS

Remind yourself that anger is a normal, human emotion and start using open body language and direct eye contact. Speak in a firm voice (but not threatening) don't attack or blame the other person. Focus on the behavior that triggered your anger. Use "I" statements, don't drag in old issues. Avoid words/statements you'll regret later. How many times have you heard someone who said something that is mean, vindictive and hurtful, or committed a violent and/ or destructive act, justify it by saying the recipient had "made" the perpetrator mad? That's an example of using blame to excuse your own bad behavior. Unfortunately, blame is like anger because it dulls one sense of empathy. It allows a person to act in a hurtful way to another human being. It isn't the act itself, but it often clears the road. This is an important point.

Experts believe, ordinary humans have inhibitions that serve as a buffer against what we know is bad behavior. Blame is not the act itself, but it either erodes or outright removes these inhibitions, often both. It's been said anger develops a thought pattern that allows the person's emotions to override his/her self-control in order to achieve an often selfish end, including sustaining dysfunctional patterns.

In addition, this may seem like an overly harsh statement, you should also realize the kind of mindset that so quickly adopts blame as a defensive posture for emotional/ego protection is exactly the same one that will put you in front of, otherwise avoidable, physical danger. People who blame others tend to overemphasize themselves while at the same time underemphasizing the negative effects of their actions. Realize something very important here; we didn't say "overemphasize the effects of others of them," we said, overemphasize themselves.

Overemphasizing the negative effects others have on them is very much a part of overemphasizing self. While one cannot state that all blamers have narcissistic personality disorder, blaming is a common behavior among those who fall somewhere on the continuum. This is among other form of dysfunction. However, one doesn't have to be dysfunctional to blame others, often it just boils down to plain old lazy and selfish.

"I've always thought of wholeness and integration as necessary myths. We're fragmented beings who cement ourselves together, but there are always cracks. Living with the cracks is part of being, well, reasonably healthy."
--Siri Hustvedt--

HAVE YOUR SUPPORTS POINT IT OUT IF YOU ARE UNAWARE

Experts believe, we grow up with anger right from the beginning of life. As a result, some persons will fly into rage about almost anything. However, anger is a common human experience and we all will encounter it. And we encounter it more often than we like to admit. Before going any further, we need to make a clear distinction between anger and feeling hurt or irritated. We all feel hurt or irritated when someone or something obstructs our needs or desires. Although experts say anger is not a true emotion. In its technical sense, anger refers to the desire to "get even with" that is, to take revenge on the cause of the hurt. The truth is, anger may be a "natural" that is, a commonly occurring social reaction to hurt and insult, yet being natural doesn't make it good for us.

As you know, "Natural," foods are commonly advertised as being healthy and good for us. But, on the other hand, poisons, for example, are also natural and poisons, by definition, are deadly. So there are far better ways to cope with hurt and insult than with anger, because anger itself act like a poison in your own heart that ultimately degrades the quality or your own life as much as it hurts the life of another person. So the first step in learning a healthy response to feelings of hurt and insult is simply to acknowledge that you feel hurt says Guide to Psychology.

Also, consider being quite open to family and friends about your condition. If they understand the condition, they may be able to tell if you are becoming ill, even if you do not realize it yourself, particularly, if you are developing an episode or mania. Rather than thinking of you as bizarre they may think of you as ill and may encourage you to get help. It has been shown that if you are taught to recognize the early stages of mania, you are more likely to seek help and treatment which may prevent a major episode developing. Your doctor or therapist may help to teach you about recognizing when to seek help. Episodes of mania or depression can be distressing for family and friends; particularly, a first episode of mania. Bizarre and odd behavior in a close relative or friend, which is out of character, can cause a lot of upset so it may help once you know the diagnosis. You may then understand that odd behavior of your friend or loved one is due to mental illness because people with mania usually do not realize they are ill. So, family and friends are often a great help in alerting a doctor or other healthcare worker if symptoms of a new episode of illness develop. Also, try to encourage the affected person to take their medication as prescribed and also to try the self-help coping technique.

"..Balancing time you spend with or without people is crucial for mental health."

--Amy E. Spiegel--

Chapter 7

MOOD SWINGS

According to the National Institute of Mental Health (NIMH), a mood swing is simply a noticeable change in one's mood or emotional state. Everybody has mood swings and they are a natural part of most people's lives. We get happy, we get sad and we have a period of feeling on top of the world, then later in the same day, we feel tired, lethargic and beaten down. Small mood swings are a part of most people's lives. However, some people's mood swings are so extreme, rapid or serious; that they interfere with that individual's functioning in everyday life. Bipolar disorder is the best example of a disorder that is characterized by mood swings, from manic to depress says NIMH, but you can, have mood swings between any two moods or emotions, sad to angry, happy to contemplative, etc. etc. says NIMH.

It's been suggested, people who are experiencing a mood swing that's been going on for more than a few weeks and is seriously affecting their friendships, relationship, school work, etc. should consider seeking professional help for the issue. A professional can help accurately diagnose the problem, and prescribe a course of treatment to reduce the mood swings.

In addition, mood swings are not a person's fault, nor can time always heal this kind of issue on its own. Without help, often times people get worse instead of better. Study has shown, mood swings can be so bad it can make it impossible for a person to go to class or work, or hang out with friends or your significant other. Denying you have mood swings especially if others bring it to your attention, isn't going to make things any better, but getting help for them can. Mood swings that aren't linked to a specific disorder generally come and go as a natural part of a person's life, or might be a part of a person's personality. While mood swings haven't been scientifically linked to many specific foods, drugs, or such, a common example is that of someone consuming a large amount of sugar and then coming down off of the "sugar high".

In all, the best way a person can identify their own mood swing triggers is to keep on the lookout for times when you've noticed your mood has changed significantly from what it was earlier in the day, and trace back your steps about what food, drinks or activities you may have engaged in. Tracking this pattern in a journal or online can help you identify things that may trigger or lead to a possible mood swing, allowing you to avoid those trigger in the future.

TALK ABOUT IT

Research suggests that neurotransmitters chemicals in the brain that help cells communicate with each other are slightly incorrect with people with bipolar disorder. This disruption causes mood swings, which can make them feel like the good or bad feelings will last forever. According to the National Institute of Mental Health (NIMH), the depression and the mania with bipolar disorder don't last forever, they fluctuate. Both depression and mania can create difficult feelings and emotions that can seem hard to escape. Depression is often reported as the most difficult aspect of bipolar because of the lingering feelings of unhappiness, despair, and disinterest make it completely unbearable compared to the exciting euphoria or mania says NIMH.

However, both can be dangerous if you lose grip of the fact that the good or bad feelings won't last. Even without treatment, therapy, and other proactive techniques; depression could lead to suicide, and mania could lead to erratic, irresponsible behavior. Both can have lasting, irreversible effects on your life if you give into the idea that there's no escape from the bad or an end to the good. The best way to protect yourself is to remind yourself (with the help of your therapist or others) that what you're going through won't last. This too will pass.

In addition, here are some tips to help protect yourself from the highest of highs and the lowest of lows: When you are in distress, talk to someone, this can be a family member or close friend. While you're talking about your problems, don't forget to listen to what he or she is telling you. They may have some good advice that can help out your situation. In moments of extreme distress, calling a professional, such as the therapist or a crisis hotline, may be in order.

Or, talking about it to your friends and family members about the problem you have identified. It may be a certain place, person or even time of day that is bothering you. Try to resolve your conflict. If it is a problem with another person, try to get the courage to discuss what is going on with the individual.

And, if you are financially stressed with a job loss set small goals toward finding employment. Also, take a small break when going through mood swings. Such as, going for a short walk and clear your head, get some fresh air or even treat yourself to a snack. It is very important to speak with your doctor if nothing else has helped. Your doctor may be able to prescribe medication, or coping skills, that may help you along the way until you can get rid of your depression and mood swings.

"Do all kids have to worry about their parents' mental health? The way society is set up, parents are supposed to be the grown-up ones and look after the kids, but a lot of times it's the other way around."

--Ruth Ozeki--

TAKE A BREAK AND SIT QUIETLY

A bad mood can ruin your whole day. Here are some techniques you can learn to help get over your mood. It is suggested that you create a list of ideas that you can pull from in difficult times. Take a break and have a cup of tea and sit quietly for 15 minutes. Keep your mind blank if you can. It's been said often the silence is enough to change your mood. Sitting quietly keeping your mind off everything and brings you back to the here and now. I particularly like having a cup of hot tea in the winter and a cold frosty in the summer. Find your own special place to gather strength such as, sitting by the ocean/river/pond/lake, visiting a mountain range, sitting or standing by a lovely garden.

In the summer, the best place for me to change my mood, is by the lake and watch the waves and the sky. I love to watch the waves come in and out. Planting my plants also gives me a boost that last all day. I've been told by others that looking up at mountains does the same for them. At the present time I don't live by any mountain ranges so I have to be thankful for the lake, and if mountains are something I what to see I can always take a vacation. Sometimes, all you need is to take five minutes to calm down to yourself. When you feel yourself getting heated, whether it's over an email exchange or an annoying situation at the market, just take five minutes to be still, focus on getting your breathing back to normal, and wait until you stop feeling angry before you return to the situation. Remember that there's no shame in taking a break and returning to situation with a more even mind.

In addition, sometimes all you need is a change in environment. Maybe you've been cooped up too long at home and need to go outside to get some fresh air. Or, maybe you've been driving from place to place all day and just need to sit down.

Whatever it is, taking a break from what you're doing can impact your mood in a positive way. Everyone does something different to get to his or her "calm place." You should experiment and find what works for you. It's been said, some people just need to take a walk to clear their minds and other people love sitting back with a warm cup of peppermint or chamomile tea. Some like to listen to jazz or classical music, or to spend a few minutes with their beloved dog or cat.

The bottom line is find whatever makes you feel the most calm and the most in control of your emotions, and find a way to go to your "happy place" whenever you're in one of your moods.

"Mental Health is measured though motivation to live; the more plans you have and the more significant they are, the healthier you are."
--Mark Brightlife--

BE CONSEQUENCE AWARE

We've all experienced moments of mood swings when our emotions push us into making, well, not the wisest choices. When we get frustrated, we often do things that aren't positive says Ken Lindner, who's a life coach, the celebrity agent to Matt Lauer and Dr. Sanjay Gupta. It is suggested, never make an important decision when you're angry, frustrated and in a bad mood when caught in the heat of the moment, Lindner says to take a step back, and evaluate the situation from a clearer place. As you know when we are in a bad mood we tend to make irrational decisions especially when we're fueled by emotions that will change our mood.

So, even if you're tempted to prove someone else wrong or have your side understood ASAP, it's suggested you make it a rule of thumb to never make a decision when you love to lash out, "cool down," and think about what it is you really want out of the choice of interaction, until you are in a better mood. Be consequence aware. Here is a quick way to re-focus on what matters and act accordingly, think about what you've invested in the situation and in yourself; time at your job building seniority, for example, how it might be affected. One poor decision made from anger of a mood swing can throw off all you've worked for and "it can take twenty years to build a reputation and five minutes to ruin it."

In addition, think about what you are doing, before you do it. Whether about a relationship you have or a personal problem, do not do anything rash during a mood swing without thinking about the results, and planning how you will do what you wish. Better yet, if you know you are in a mood swing, wait until you have recovered. We know some consequences can be server, but sometimes it's worth it, that's what you have to decide for yourself.

Make the right decision to avoid rash decisions because it can lead to a bad choice. Also, don't do something out of feelings in the moment of a mood swing, take some days to be sure about what you want, and wait until you are calm and relaxed before you make the final decision and do something about it; it's a good idea to confide in someone and get some opinions on what you could do. Do not over-think everything this can be easily done if you are a logical thinker. Don't get nervous at small things that require small decisions that will not affect your life further.

Lastly, you should make sure it is important enough to you to the point that you would allow the thoughts to rent space in your head. Keep in mind, over-thinking everything can cause stress, which is very bad for you and your mood. So trust yourself and keep it moving.

Note: Just remember, sometimes decisions you make while experiencing a mood swing cannot be reverted, and you will have to live with the consequences.

"May your choices reflect your hopes, not your fears."
--Nelson Mandela--

POSITIVE SELF-TALK

Self-talk is the "little voice inside your head". It is what you tell yourself about yourself, or about a situation. Self-talk can be positive, like when you tell yourself "I can do this" to help you get through something you're nervous about. Or, it can be negative, like when you tell yourself "I'm so stupid" and beat yourself up about a mistake you've made. Self-talk has a huge influence on your feelings and your mood and can make you feel better or worse about any given situation. If your self-talk tends to be negative, you probably spend a lot more time feeling angry (at yourself or at others) than someone who self-talks is positive. Is your glass half-empty or half-full? How you answer this question about positive thinking may reflect your outlook on life, your attitude toward yourself, and whether you're optimistic or pessimistic, and it may even affect your health.

Some studies show that personality traits like optimism and pessimism can affect many areas of your health and well-being. The positive thinking that typically comes with optimism is a key part of effective stress management. And effective stress management is associated with many health benefits, and if you tend to be pessimistic, don't lose hope. Moreover, it's been said positive self-talk can help you relax during a mood swing or change. When you are thinking negative thoughts that causes your mood to shift, try shifting your thoughts to positive.

Now, I know it may be easier said than done, but positive thinking doesn't mean that you keep your head in the sand and ignore life's less pleasant situations. Positive thinking just means that you approach unpleasantness in a more positive and productive way. You think the best is going to happen, not the worst. Positive thinking often starts with self-talk. Self-talk is said to be the endless steams of unspoken thoughts that run through your head. These automatic thoughts can be positive or negative. Some of your self-talk comes from logic and reason. Other self-talk may take place from misconceptions that you create because of lack of information. If the thoughts that run through your head are mostly negative your outlook on life is more likely pessimistic. If your thoughts are mostly positive, you're likely an optimist, someone who practices positive thinking.

It's unclear why people who engage in positive thinking experience these health benefits. One theory is that having a positive outlook enables you to cope better with stressful situations, which reduces the harmful health effects of stress on your body. It's also thought that positive and optimistic people tend to live healthier life style; they get more physical activity, follow a healthier diet, and don't smoke or drink alcohol in excess.

"It's never overacting to ask for what you want and need."
--Amy Poehler--

HEALTHY SLEEPING HABITS

Experts believe healthy sleep habits can make a big difference in your quality of life and can set your mood for the day. Having healthy sleep habit is often referred to as having good "sleep hygiene". Research suggest in order to maintain a health mood you will have to stick to the same bedtime and wake up time, even on the weekends because this helps to regulate your body's clock and could help you fall asleep and stay asleep for the night.

It is suggested to practice a relaxing bedtime ritual. A relaxing, routine (ritual) activity the night before bedtime that is conducted away from bright lights helps separate your sleep time from activities that can cause excitement, stress or anxiety which can make it more difficult to fall asleep, get sound and deep sleep or remain asleep. Avoid naps especially in the afternoon. Some people say sleeping during the day interrupts their sleep at night. Power napping may help you get through the day, and for some people it does not affect their sleep at night. But if you find that you can't fall asleep at bedtime, eliminating short cat naps may help. Another way to ensure you get the proper rest at night is to exercise daily. Vigorous exercise is best, but even light exercise is better than no activity. Exercise at any time of day, but not at the expense of your sleep. Design your sleep environment to establish the conditions you need for sleep. It's been suggested that your bedroom should be cool between 60-67 degrees and your bedroom should also be free from any noise that can disturb your sleep.

Finally, your bedroom should be free from any light. So check your room for noises or other distractions. This includes a bed partner's sleep disruptions such as snoring. Consider using blackout curtains, eye shades, ear plugs, "white noise" machines, humidifiers, fans and other devices.

If you can, sleep on a comfortable mattress and make sure your mattress is comfortable and supportive.

In addition, research shows that most people will agree that a lack of sleep causes them to be tired the next day; many don't realize there are other effects on the body as well such as mood swings. While some of these problems might not seem too sever, others can prove to be far more dangerous than simple items to look over. In fact, researchers have documented some of the dangers you might encounter, if you aren't sleeping. One of the most common things that a lack of sleep causes is anger issues. While you might think that you are simple cranky naturally, the problem could be from a total lack of sleep.

Studies have shown that this also causes impatience and sudden mood swings as well. In some cases, you might find that it changes your overall personality. In addition to this, your immune system will begin to suffer as well. While you are losing sleep, your body can't regenerate and refuel parts of your body when it is needed. This causes your immune system to continue working in overdrive and soon, you become more susceptible to flue and other illnesses you might have normally would not have gotten.

"I mind the unmindful, but I mind my own mind too. Mine your mind, and mine the minds of others. Mind..You are mine!"
--Justin K. McFarlane Beau—

NUTRITION

As was previously stated, nutrition is another vital component to mood management. Sugar, alcohol, medication and caffeine are just the things that can sharply increase or decrease mood affects.

Research suggests that certain foods affect mood for better or worse. Dietary changes can trigger chemical and physiological changes within the brain that alter our behavior and emotions. "Most people understand the link between what they eat and their physical health," says registered dietitian Elizabeth Somer, "but the link between what you eat and your mood, your energy, how you sleep, and how well you think is much more immediate." "What you eat or don't eat for breakfast will have at least a slight effect by mid-afternoon and what you're eating all day will have a huge impact today and down the road."

In addition, dietary experts suggest, getting too little iron can spell depression, fatigue, and inattention. Iron-rich foods include red meat, egg yolk, dried fruit, beans, liver, and artichokes. Scientists have also found that insufficient thiamine can cause "introversion, inactivity, fatigue, decreased self-confidence, and poor mood, "according to a recent report published in the Darmouth Undergraduate Journal of Science. Thiamine abounds in cereal gains, pork, yeast, cauliflower, and eggs, and getting enough increases well-being, sociability, and your overall energy level.

Also, equally important is folic acid because it helps fend off depression. In addition, green veggies, oranges, grapefruit, nuts, sprouts, and whole-wheat bread are good sources. It's been said you can eat too much fat. That bag of potato chips isn't good for your waistline or your mood.

In fact, greasy choices, particularly those high in saturated fat are linked to both depression and dementia says Somer. And, a large, high-fat meal will almost instantly make you feel sluggish. "It takes a lot of work for our bodies to digest fat," Gans says. "And since there's more work going on, you're obviously going to end up feeling tired."

""Everybody struggles with this stuff, you know. With social discomfort and grief and fitting in. People with syndromes, people with disorders, people with diagnoses, and without People who would be classified as neurotypical, idiots and geniuses, maids and doctors. Nobody's got it all figured out."
--Jael McHenry--

CHANGING YOUR PERSPECTIVE

First, you have to stop assuming the worst. The facts show if you have frequent mood swings, then you may be the kind of person who always assumes that the worst possible thing will happen in a given situation. For example, you may be waiting to hear back from a job and assume you didn't get it after a day has passed.

Or, your mother may say that she has something to tell you and you assume this means that she's deadly ill. Well, this kind of thinking is likely to lead you to feeling very angry and upset for little or no reason. Instead of assuming the worst that can happen, think about all of the scenarios that are possible. This will help you realize that the worse is not likely to happen, and there's no point in getting all upset until and know more. You can think about the worst that can happen and prepare for it, just in case, but avoid dwelling on it or letting it ruin your mood.

Also, being able to see something through the eyes of someone else takes practice. You can experiment with the following techniques to see which works well for you. Research shows if you want to understand another perspective, resist the urge to debate. Instead, consider paraphrasing and repeating back what you've heard, mirror it back to the person so he/she knows whether you understood the points the way they intended. Be sure to use the words you actually heard, or reasonable paraphrasing.

And, watch your tone of voice and work to avoid overstating or generalizing what they said, first check to determine if you heard them correctly, to validate that you were listening.

Then ask for a chance to express your side of things. You can't go wrong.

"Stigma's power lies in silence. The silence that persists when discussion and action should be taking place. The silence one imposes on another for speaking up on a taboo subject, branding them with a label until they are rendered mute or preferably unheard."

--M.B. Dallocchio--

SHIFT YOUR FEELINGS

Most of the time, you can avoid these common emotional traps and improve your emotional health, attitudes, and self-esteem. Researchers have documented one method of shifting emotion which is called the Bares model. The Bares model show you how to be aware of all your emotions, and accept them all without judgment, recognize that you control your attitudes and behaviors, express true emotions that will allow you to shift negatives consciously. Once you recognize an emotion you are feeling, you may decide that this particular emotion isn't helpful for you in that moment or circumstance. This is not to deny an emotion or to avoid processing it later if necessary.

Rather, it's about making a conscious decision to shift your feeling state. Positive feeling states are associated with healthier bodies, improved thinking, and enhanced decision-making capabilities. Intentionally invoking a positive feeling state can enhance our ability to function in our lives.

On the other hand, when we are negative, frustrated, or angry, we tend to lose focus and become less affective. How do you shift to a more positive state? It's been suggested to actually re-experience the positive feeling state and experience it in your body (not just visualizing it or talking about it). In less than a minute, you can shift an emotion, change your physiology, and become more effective and happier.

The facts show your body is capable of responding in just a few breaths. A study conducted by the Institute of Heart Math examined the impact of positive emotions on physical and mental functioning. The Institute asserts that our capacity to self-generate a positive emotional state and quickly shift to a physiologically coherent mode at will can be developed and refined.

The study goes on to suggest the physiological coherence is a natural human state that can occur spontaneously during positive emotional experiences and sleep, but maintaining episodes are generally rare. Using positive emotion to drive the coherent mode allows it to emerge naturally, which makes it easier to maintain this positive state for longer periods, even during work and other activities. So let's start shifting our feelings to a positive state today.

"A person is also mentally weak by the quantity of time he spends to sneak peek into others lives to devalue and degrade the quality of his own life."

--Anuj Somany--

Chapter 8

RACING THOUGHTS

According to the National Institute of Mental Health (NIMH), racing thoughts mean you are thinking in overdrive. Racing thoughts are not just "thinking fast," They are thoughts that just won't be quite; they can be in the background of other thoughts or take over a person's consciousness; they can run around in the sufferer's head like a carousel gone out of control says NIMH. Before anyone knew anything about bipolar disorder, it was called this sensation "racy brain." Some people say thoughts and music zoom through their head so fast that sometimes they want to scream.

And, if it was going on at bedtime, it could take them an hour or more of concentrating on word games to get to sleep. Experts believe the components of racing thoughts can include music, snatches of conversation from movies or television or books, one's own voice or other voices repeating a phrase or sentences again and again, or even rhythms of pressure without any "sound" in the thought.

According to the National Institute of Mental Health, the phenomenon called racing thoughts is distinct from "hearing voices," which is a symptom of schizophrenia, schizoaffective disorder, severe mania or other psychotic disorders. Racing thoughts can also be a symptom of mania, hypomania or a mixed episode, but unlike some other symptoms of these moods, they can also occur with depression or an anxiety disorder. It's been said sometimes racing thoughts are accompanied by a pounding heart or pounding pulses, including drumming in the ears. While racing thoughts are most commonly described in people with bipolar disorder, they are also common with anxiety disorders, such as OCD and psychiatric disorders such as attention deficit hyperactivity disorder says NIMH.

In addition, a study has shown, racing thoughts are also associated with use of amphetamines, sleep deprivation, as well as hypothyroidism. It is evidence showing racing thoughts may be experienced as background or take over a person's consciousness. Thoughts, music, and voices might be zooming thought one's mind as they jump logically from one to the next. Experts believe there also might be a repetitive pattern of voices or of pressure without any associate "sound". It is a very overwhelming and irritating feeling, and can result in losing track of time.

Generally, racing thoughts are described by an individual who has had an episode as an event where the mind uncontrollable brings up random thoughts and memories and switches between them very quickly. Sometimes they are related, as one thought leads to another, other times they seem completely random. The facts show a person suffering from an episode of racing thoughts has no control over his or her train of thought and it stops them from focusing on one topic or prevents sleeping. Racing thoughts, also referred to as "racing mind", may prevent a person from falling asleep. Chronic sleep apnea and prolonged disturbed sleep patterns may also induce racing thoughts.

WRITING

The medical profession believes racing thoughts can be a symptom of mental illness; they are not specific to any particular illness. Experts believe, racing thoughts can occur during anxiety states, panic attacks, and during the "manic" phase of bipolar disorders, as well as during drug intoxication states. You need to learn more about why you are having racing thoughts before you can know if there is any medication that can help you with them. I suggest a visit to your local psychiatrist so that you can be properly diagnosed. The psychiatrist will be in the best position to know what medications or coping skills might be helpful to you if you are experiencing a clinical problem.

In addition, one coping skill I would suggest is writing, whether it's a journal blog, or creative writing, the act of writing will engage your mind and reduce the power of racing thoughts. Writing out the thoughts can be easy. It starts with trying to write out any of these thoughts on some type of paper or journal. Something that few people realize is that your mind tries very hard to remember things, especially before sleep. The mind also doesn't worry about remembering things when it knows there is a note of them somewhere. Racing thoughts may occur because your brain is trying to remember the thoughts you can control, so write them out on a piece of paper to give your brain a break and to help you relax.

Also, try writing down your worries-earlier in the day. For about 10 to 15 minutes a day, "Write down what's on your mind at an earlier time and what you're doing about it, "says Sherman Silberman, author of The Insomnia Workbook: A Comprehensive Guide to Getting the Sleep You Need. To kick-start your worry session, she suggests simply asking yourself, "What are the things that come to my mind when I'm lying in bed at night?" If a worrying thought comes up right before bed, you "can mentally check it off," and either say to yourself "I've dealt with that," or "I'm dealing with it, "she says. This usually helps to create a "sense of relief. Lastly, avoid writing up your list before bedtime Sherman says, because you want to have enough separation from your thoughts at night.

"If your love for another person doesn't include loving yourself then your love is incomplete."
--Shannon L. Alder--

PHYSICAL ACTIVITY

Researchers have documented things like running, swimming, basketball; weight lifting, etc. When you engage your body it will eventually engage your mind. As your body becomes fatigued your mind will become more consumed by that than anything else. It's been said having racing thoughts can be disturbing and frightening because it creates a sense of being out of control. But having racing thoughts does not mean you're out of control or crazy. What it does mean is you are anxious and that your stress levels are elevated.

According to the National Institute of Mental Health (NIMH) anxiety and racing thoughts just go hand and hand but it is manageable. Jogging is an outstanding tool for tiring the mind. Fitness doesn't just tire muscles. It makes your brain more relaxed as well, by releasing chemicals that provide a relaxation/calming effect. So exercising and/ or going for a good run is incredibly valuable. Also, if you can't intensely exercise, walk. Walking provides a great deal of sensory distraction (new sights, sounds, and smells anywhere you walk, even if you're in your own apartment) and provides a bit of extra blood flow that may be useful for calming your body.

Moreover, give yourself a task; find something you can do for a while as your mind continues to race. Tasks give you something to focus on so you don't worry too much about your thoughts racing. Studies have shown if you try to stop it, you'll actually make it worse. Instead, give yourself something to do that puts your focus on something that doesn't requires as much thoughts, like catching up on your favorite website. That focus will help to ease your mind back into reality and should slow your thoughts down considerably. All of those tips are about reducing the length of time you suffer from racing thoughts.

Remember, you cannot simply stop them immediately because the more you try to fight them away, the more likely the voices will continue. The only proven way to stop your racing thoughts is to stop your anxiety. I've helped people with racing thoughts keep their anxiety from coming back during my 14 years in the mental health field by learning more about their anxiety and using coping technique found in this book.

"Self-discipline is the ability to organize your behavior over time in the service of specific goals."
--Nathaniel Branden---

CLEARING YOUR THOUGHTS

It's been said once our mind is cleared, we start experiencing inner peace. Experts believe, the most important thing to do to clear your mind is to concentrate. Concentration, meditation and the development of inner detachment help clear the mind of thoughts, making room for inner peace. There is no instant inner peace says Psych Central. In order to attain and enjoy inner peace, work and effort are required, but not everyone is willing to invest the necessary time and energy into this project. One exercise that will help your concentration is meditation, you use the skills gained thought the development of the power of concentration, in order to free your mind of thoughts. There are many forms of meditation, which all help clear the mind of thoughts, and which ultimately lead to the ability to meditate without thoughts.

The second way to clear your thoughts is detachment. Without some inner detachment there is no inner peace. You need to learn not to be affected easily by what people what or do, and not let your emotions rule your life. I am not taking about being indifferent and uncaring. But you can be compassionate, helpful and full of love, and at the same time display inner detachment. It is a mental attitude which leads to common sense, better judgment, more understanding and inner peace. You can find a lot of information, instructions and exercises for developing the skills leading to inner peace in this book on meditation.

Lastly, focus on the positive. When you're lying in bed worrying, it helps to turn to more positive thoughts. You can "focus on good memories and happy events." Extensive studies say that, when you determinately decide to change your mind, you cause physical changes to your brain. Providing the change is in a positive direction, this is fantastic news.

Study has shown this can also involve a change in behavior to eliminate a compulsive pattern, take your life back form an addiction, or heal your relationship with money or food, a person you love or a difficult boss or colleague. Change and healing are about reshaping your mindset in a particular area of your life. You can make this a conscious process, where shifts in your thoughts, attitude and beliefs rewire current problematic emotional circuits.

It has been scientifically shown that the brain is structurally altered by changes in your behavior patterns. You can conquer toxic thanking patterns and old limiting beliefs by conscious shifts in your views, having a new vision, and reframing problems. It is safe to say, you get to consciously choose what you will create or change.

"If I don't write to empty my mind, I go mad."
--Lord Byron--

READ

Yes, read a book, this simple technique is useful because it tends to occupy your inner voice. Research shows if you are reading and following the story it's much more difficult to slip back into other thoughts at the same time. One of the best choices for this type of bedtime reading is an exciting book that you've read before where you know the ending. The cliff hangers have less impact, but the story is just as engaging and just as far from your own worries as it ever was. Trust yourself to know which kind of book keeps you awake and which one puts you to sleep. Some people read Stephen King to get to sleep, but it's still often better to enjoy a King reread than to dive into a new one where you don't know how it comes out yet. Be careful because for some people this has the opposite effect, making them more awake, especially if you are reading an extremely exciting book. Are you stressed out? Try picking up a paperback.

Research conducted in 2009 at Mindlab International at the University of Sussex showed that reading was the most effective way to overcome stress, beating out old favorites such as listening to music, enjoying a cup of tea or coffee and even taking a walk, The Telegraph reported when the findings were released. It took the study participants just six minutes to relax (which was measured by evaluating heart rate and muscle tension) once they started turning pages. "It really doesn't matter what book you read, by losing yourself in a thoroughly engrossing book you can escape from the worries and stresses of the everyday world and spend a while exploring the domain of the author's imagination," study researcher Dr. David Lewis told The Telegraph.

In addition, self-help books might actually help you help yourself. A study published earlier this year in the journal PLOS ONE showed that reading self-help books (also called bibliotgherapy), combined with support sessions on how to use them, was linked with lower levels of depression after a year, compared to patients who received typical treatments. It was found this had a really significant clinical impact and the findings are very encouraging, study author Christopher Williams of the University of Glasgow told the BBC. "Depression zaps people's motivation and makes it hard to believe changes are possible."

Also, self-help books could even work in case of severe depression as well as help slow down your racing thoughts. According to a University of Manchester meta-analysis published earlier this year, people who experience racing thoughts can benefit from "low-intensity interventions," including self-help books and interactive websites, as much or more than those who experience other mental health illness.

"Can you imagine how your life would be if you couldn't talk?"

--Naoki Higashida--

BREAKING THOUGHTS INTO SMALLER PIECES

You want to know how to stop and keep scary thoughts away. According to the National Institute of Mental Health (NIMH) as long as you have anxiety you're going to be prone to these types of scary thoughts. Anxiety changes brain chemistry, and makes it easier for the mind to focus on the negative. You're not only more likely to have scary thoughts when you have anxiety you're also more likely to focus on the thoughts. Having the thoughts can cause more anxiety, and ultimately have more scary thoughts in the future. That's a problem, so until you control your anxiety, you're going to need to find ways to avoid worrying about the thought as much.

Again, try writing the thoughts down, for reasons not quite clear, the mind is more likely to stop focusing on something scary when it has it written down in a permanent place. When these thoughts are distressing you, write the thought down in a journal. That will help you stop focusing on it as much.

In addition, you're also going to need to accept the thoughts when they occur. While they may distress you, the more you try to fight them the worse they can become. It's in your best interests to be okay with the fact that you have the thoughts, because you know you have anxiety and these thoughts are going to happen. You can also think of the purpose of the thoughts; some psychologists use a form of exposure therapy to reduce these thoughts. To do this, you need to focus on the thoughts on purpose until it stops bothering you. Purposely have the scary thoughts as often as possible until it no longer cause you to be as worried. Often this is best complete in the presence of an expert to calm you when you feel distressed.

And, anything that distracts you from the thought can be valuable as well, especially if it's positive in nature. Consider funny shows on television, podcasts or calling a friend. In the end, when we face the thoughts, we face the feelings behind the thoughts and eventually you will become familiar with the feelings and no longer fell anxious which in turn will resolve some of your racing thoughts.

"My sadness is beautiful. It infuses everything I do. It is at the core of my identity and always has been, just as happiness is in some people. I refuse to be told that it's a flaw. I will not mute it with medications for the sake of society. I will hold it close to me and celebrate it rightfully while the rest of the world fails to see it for what it is and it will be their loss."

--Ashly Lorenzana--

DEVELOPING A DAILY LIST

If you're like a lot of people, you use a daily to-do list and you may even check some things off each day, but you may be making a mistake that many people make that cause a huge problem not only in terms of productivity, but also in the fundamental way you organize your thoughts. Don't feel bad because it's a common a mistake, and I'm here to help you fix it, considering this question for a moment. What does your daily to-do list contain? Is it sufficiently broken down into manageable tasks and task only? Can you realistically complete those tasks in a maximum of a couple of hours each? Here are some helpful hints that are suggested on how to construct a proper daily to-do list.

First, a daily to-do list should be composed of small tasks that don't take more than a couple of hours at most to complete. Otherwise, they have no place on the list. This is where a lot of people go wrong. Study has shown most people use daily to-do lists as a reminder of the things they need to work on, but the use of the list ends there. They fail to separate the large projects of their list from the small tasks they need to accomplish in the first place. The result is often a major short-term focus, and is a huge reason why a lot of people in this world fail to think in a proactive fashion. Most people think one day at a time, and never a step ahead. You see, by not separating out your long-term goals and projects onto other forms of productivity documentation, the only list you'll ever have is your daily list, which at this point is only a reminder of things to work on. It's not being used in productive fashion to help you achieve your goals.

In addition, you may ask yourself, what is the best way to diffuse a racing mind? Although a simple solution, it actually can be very helpful to make a list. It is best to set aside some time in the afternoon or early evening, several hours from bedtime, to sit and write down the issues in your life that might lead to stress. These may include incomplete home or work tasks, family stress, health concerns, financial problems, and a variety of other stressors. Specify these concerns. By writing them down, you no longer have to devote mental energy to keeping track of them. As part of this, you may even write down action points, any ideas you have to reduce or eliminate the source of stress. Why is making a list helpful? This process orders your thoughts, and helps you to recognize, organize, and articulate what is leading you to feel stress. By supplementing this with an action plan, you will decrease your stress because you have identified ways to make this better.

Also, you no longer have to worry about remembering these things. If you can set aside time each day to review the list, you will have to schedule a time to address these concerns. Then, if the thoughts come to mind as you are trying to fall asleep, you simply tell yourself, "I have written this down on my list and I will address it tomorrow when I have my time to review it." You then disengage from the anxiety, not dwelling on the thought, and let it go.

"Breathe, Relax. This too shall pass."
--Lee Horbachewski--

SUPPORT/GROUP THERAPY

Racing thoughts can be very difficult to manage on your own. If racing thoughts are interfering with your life, you may want to consider attending psychotherapy. Through psychotherapy, you can work with a mental health specialist to develop ways to manage your racing thoughts. Your therapist may also recommend that you attend group therapy. Through group therapy, you can expect to meet with a facilitator plus other clients who are dealing with the same or similar issues. Group therapy can help you to overcome feelings of loneliness while sharing experiences and exploring coping techniques and others who can relate to your symptoms. Group therapy may also provide you with tips and techniques to get past racing thoughts.

In addition to professional help, it may also be useful to have a trusted friend or family member to turn to when racing thoughts seem unbearable. Sometimes just having a person to talk with can assist you in slowing down your thoughts. In addition, support groups bring together people facing similar issues, whether that's illness, relationship problems or major life changes. Members of support groups often share experiences and advice and it can be helpful just getting to talk with other people who are in the same boat. While not everyone wants or needs support beyond that offered by family and friends, you may find it helpful and rewarding to turn to other outside your immediate circle.

Also, a support group can help you cope better and feel less isolated as you make connections with others facing similar challenges. A support group shouldn't replace your standard medical care, but it can be a valuable resource to help you cope.

Regardless of format, in a support group, you'll find people with problems similar to yours. Members of a support group typically share their personal experiences and offer one another emotional comfort and moral support. They may also offer practical advice and tips to help you cope with your situation.

Study has shown the benefits of participating in support groups may include: Feeling less lonely, isolate or judge; you gain a sense of empowerment and control, improving your coping skills and sense of adjustment, talking openly and honestly about your feelings. It helps to reduce distress, depression or anxiety while developing a clearer understanding of what to expect with your situation. You will also get the opportunity to compare notes about resources, such as doctors, websites, medication side-effects, and alternative medicine.

"Dishonoring what we feel is an epidemic that has us self-medicating as a culture and trying to numb ourselves."
--Abiola Abrams--

FOCUS

Every single second, our brains take in an incredible amount of information 11 million bits of information per second to be exact says Joseph Cardillo, Ph.D, writes in his book, Can I Have Your Attention? How to Think Fast, Find Your Focus, and Sharpen your Concentration? But we actually pay attention to about 40 bits. Which is still a lot particularly, if you're trying to complete or even start a task. So finding focus can seem like a farfetched accomplishment. Especially in "today's 24/7 world," focus is something we're sorely lacking, according to Christine Louise Hohlbaum. But, focus isn't all or nothing. It's not something we either have or don't have. It's a skill that we can develop and practice makes perfect (or at least good enough).

Below, various experts on attention and focus share their favorite tips for finding focus in our distraction overloaded day and age. For example, create a gadget-free zones, Hohlbaum recommended. "While our gadgets are meant to save us time, many times they actually waste it." For many of us, cell phones have become another accessory and this can be detrimental to our attention spans (and our relationships). Hohlbaum suggested establishing areas like your living room or your kitchen table as gadget-free zone. When you're on the computer, close your windows on the screen, she said. "If you have 20 applications open at one time, chances are you are toggling from one to the next." Keep only the windows open you need for the task at hand. Like Hohlbaum said, this isn't just a blessing for your brain capacity "but it also uses less computer memory."

Also, get outside. If you mind is meandering, according to Lucy Jo Palladino, PhD, psychologist and author of find Your Focus Zone: An Effective New Plan to Defeat Distraction and Overload, a "quick walk outdoors" is an effective short break. Like Hohlbaum said, many of us spend a lot of time in unnatural settings, such as office and cubicles. Instead, get outside and, as Palladino suggested, take "some deep breaths" while focused on a beautiful object, preferably or nature a plant, a flower, the sky outside your window." Just, "Before you leave, write down what time you'll return to work, and make a commitment to it."

"Make sure your priorities line up with your values."
--Michael Barbarulo--

PROGRESSIVE MUSCLE RELAXATION

According to fitness experts on breathing techniques, progressive muscle relaxation, it is very easy to learn, all you have to do is bring yourselves in a pleasant state of relaxation by progressively tensing and then relaxing different muscle groups through your entire body. Here is an example of the proper technique for progressive muscle relaxation.

Example:

First, relaxing your arms and close your eyes, if you like it, and guide your attention to your right arm. At first just try to perceive your right arm and hand, becoming aware of the feelings and sensations in this area of your body. Notice the places at which your arm touches your body or the armrest.

Next, make a fist with your right hand, hold the tension for a moment, and be aware of the feelings of tension in your right forearm and in the right hand. And now let go again, relax and soften your hand and your forearm. Try to notice, how your musculature is relaxing completely by itself. You don't have to force or to do anything actively, accept your experience just as it is. Soften and relax your fingers, be aware of the decreasing tension in the thumb, in the forefinger, middle finger, in the ring finger and in the small finger.

Once again, make a fist with your right hand. Hold the tension for a moment, hold it, hold it, and now let go again, be aware of the different feelings of tension and relaxation. This is a wonderful technique that can be done every day. My groups love it.

Remember to be careful. Be careful not to hurt yourself while tensing your muscles. You should never feel intense or shooting pain while completing this exercise.

Make the muscle tension deliberate, yet gentle. If you have problems with pulled muscles, broken bones, or any medical issues that would hinder physical activity, consult your doctor first.

> *"Obstacles are those frightful things you see when you take your eyes off your goal."*
>
> *--Henry Ford--*

SHUT OFF YOUR BRAIN BEFORE BEDTIME

For many of us, as soon as it's time for bed, the brain begins buzzing. We might experience racing thoughts or a thought or two that keeps growling at us when we have something on our mind. If continued, those thoughts can turn into worry thoughts about not being able to function the next day because you slept poorly. It can become a vicious cycle. While there's "no button to push" to deactivate our thoughts, of course, we can "create the right associations" to help us sleep well, say Lawrence Epstein, M.D., chief medical officer of Sleep Health Centers and instructor in medicine at Harvard University.

Below, Dr. Epstein and sleep specialist Stephanie Silberman, Ph.D, share their insight on how to quiet your worries and sleep well.

First, you must realize sleep is essential. For many of us, sleep is the last thing on our minds when it comes to living healthfully. And sleep will be the first thing to get sacrificed if we're pressed for time. Once you realize that sleep is vital to your life, he says, you can work on sleeping well.

1. Have a regular sleep schedule. Getting up and going to bed at the same time is the key to good sleep. In fact. Dr. Epstein says that "the greatest promoter of being able to sleep is being in sync with your internal clock" or your circadian rhythms.

2. Crate a pre-sleep routine. Along with a consistent sleep/wake schedule, winding down before bed is one of the best ways to get your sleep back on track. As Siilberman says, it's "very hard to shut down your brain or quiet anxious or worrying thoughts when you're on the go before bedtime." You want to separate your day

from the nighttime, he says. Also, "Our body craves routine and likes to know what's coming," says Dr. Epstein, also co-author of The Harvard Medical School Guide to a good Night's sleep. By creating a pre-sleep ritual, you're establishing a clear association between certain activities and sleep.

Lastly, for example, if you read before heading to bed, your body knows that reading at night signals sleep time. If you take a warm bath before bed every night, your body recognizes that it's time to slow down and relax. Also, Silberman suggest listening to calming music, stretching or doing relaxation exercises. And if you're watching TV before bed, make sure it's at least a relaxing program and not something like the news, she adds. The goal of this pre-sleep routine is to relax your body and prime it for sleep, Dr. Epstein says. So if you're going to bed at 10 or 11 p.m., "set aside 30 minutes or an hour for pre-sleep time," he says.

"A healthy society begins with healthy individuals."
--Sabina Nore--

Chapter 9

OBESSIVE THOUGHTS/BEHAVIORS
Obsessive-Compulsive Disorder (OCD)

It's normal, on occasion, to go back and double-check that the iron is unplugged or your car is locked. If you suffer from Obsessive Compulsive Disorder (OCD), obsessive thoughts and compulsive behaviors become so excessive they interfere with your daily life. No matter what you do; you can't seem to shake them. But help is available. With treatment and self-help strategies, you can break free of the unwanted thoughts and irrational urges and take back control of your life.

According to the American Psychiatric Association, Diagnostic and Statistical Manual of Mental Disorders, Obsessive Compulsive Disorder (OCD) is an anxiety disorder characterized by uncontrollable, unwanted thoughts and repetitive, ritualized behaviors you feel compelled to perform. If you have OCD, you probably recognize that you have obsessive thoughts or urge to repeat yourself. For example, you may check the stove twenty times to make sure it's really turned off, wash your hands until they're scrubbed raw, or drive around for hours to make sure that the bump you heard while driving wasn't a person you ran over. Obsessive are involuntary, seemingly uncontrollable thoughts, images or impulses that occur over and over again in your mind. You don't want to have these ideas but you can't stop them.

Unfortunately, these obsessive thoughts are often disturbing and distracting. Compulsions are behaviors or rituals that you feel driven to act out again and again. Usually, compulsions are performed in an attempt to make obsessions go away says National Institute of Mental Health.

For example, if you're afraid of contamination, you might develop elaborate cleaning rituals. However, the relief never last. In fact, Studies has shown the obsessive thoughts usually come back stronger. And the compulsive behaviors often end up causing anxiety themselves as they become more demanding and time-consuming. OCD compulsions can begin in one area of a person's life and spread to others, with the same behavior patterns such as wasting and cleaning, counting, checking, demanding reassurances, performing the same action repeatedly, and orderliness.

TALK TO YOUR DOCTOR

Tell your doctor all of the symptoms you are experiencing that you think may be indicative of obsessive compulsive disorder. He'll need to have complete and accurate information in order to make an informed diagnosis. Also, talk to your doctor about the severity of your symptoms, including, how much they interfere with you daily life. The severity of the symptoms is very important because it will have a large bearing on the treatment that is ultimately selected for you.

And, ask your doctor to explain the long-term prospects for people who suffer from OCD and any potential side effects of the condition or medication. It's been said it makes most people feel more secure and confident about dealing with a disorder if they know what to expect from it. Also, go over treatment options with your doctor. You should find out about what medications are available to treat OCD as well as whether you are a good candidate for cognitive therapy. If cognitive therapy is selected, you should get your doctor or friend to recommend the therapist he/she thinks is the best in the area or on the internet.

Moreover, Experts believe most people with OCD benefit from a form of therapy called cognitive-behavioral therapy or CBT; The facts show, about 75% of people who participate in CBT have few OCD symptoms. Cognitive-behavioral therapy is given by a mental health professional such as a psychiatrist or psychologist/therapist. In this type of therapy, you work with the professional to identify your obsessions and compulsions. Once your unhealthy thoughts and behaviors are identified, the professional will introduce a number of techniques designed to help you challenge your thoughts and learn new ways of coping with anxiety and compulsions. One type of CBT will slowly exposes you to things that trigger your obsessive thoughts, while helping you develop the skills you need to resist your compulsions. Although CBT is usually a short-term treatment, practicing the skills you learn both during and after treatment can help you manage your symptoms for a long time to come. It's been suggested to attend support groups because it will help you to know you are not alone. Anxiety disorder support groups, including ones for OCD, are a great way to share your experiences and learn from the experiences of others.

Or, Self-help book (such as this one) can help you during and after treatment, there are some things you can do on your own to help keep you feeling better. Such as, regular exercise, eating well, managing stress, spending time with friends and family, spirituality, and monitoring your use of alcohol and other drugs can help keep anxiety from getting worse or coming back. Again, talking to your doctor, asking question, and feeling in charge of your own health are also very important. Always talk to your doctor about what you're doing on your own to help your OCD.

"You gain strength, courage and confidence by every experience in which you really stop to look fear in the face."
--Eleanor Roosevelt--

HUMOR

I feel laughter is the best medicine for any illness. Humor is a virus to us. According to research the sound of roaring laughter is far more contagious than any cough, sniffle, or sneeze and when laughter is shared it binds people together and increases happiness and intimacy. Laughter also triggers healthy physical changes in the body. Some would say it's a great workout for the organs in your body. Because when you laugh it shakes you up in the inside.

Also, humor and laughter strengthen your immune system, boost your energy, diminish pain, and protect you from the damaging effects of stress. Best of all, this priceless medicine is fun, free, and easy to us. Obsessive-compulsive disorder is often portrayed as a quirky, curtsey, bothersome at most, illness. This couldn't be further from the truth. According to the National Institute of Mental Health, OCD is a potentially devastating neurologically based anxiety disorder with the ability to destroy lives. There is nothing funny about it. But that doesn't mean we can't use humor when dealing with OCD. While there is nothing amusing about having it, the situations that often arise from dealing with the disorder can be downright funny, what OCD sufferer doesn't have a story or two to tell that would be sure to make us laugh as well as themselves?

In addition, humor is your secret weapon; it is one of the most powerful weapons in the arsenal of OCD fighters. (It's not bad against other life problems, either.) It's a simple thing, one you can't buy or make, although you can encourage its development. It's something no one can give you, but others can foster in your humor. If you don't have a sense of humor, get one. Happily, most people who have OCD do seem to enjoy well-developed abilities to see the funnier aspects and absurdities of their condition. And this doesn't mean that it isn't at the same time, terrible. No one will tell you that OCD is fun, but it can be funny. Even at its most horrible, it can be funny. As a group, people who have OCD tend to be bright and creative. Many possess excellent senses of humor. So think of your sense of humor as your "secret weapon" against despair, hopelessness and OCD itself. As OCD seems to affect bright, creative people, you may as well turn some of your mental energies and talent away from obsessive worries and toward the humor in everyday life, particularly yours.

Humor, generally, is good for your mental health, your physical health, and (assuming it's not cruel or sarcastic) your relationships. Try to fit as much of it as you can into your life as I do.

"For every minute you are angry you lose sixty seconds of happiness."
--Ralph Waldo Emerson--

PEGGYBACKING REALITY/REALITY TESTING

Imagine that your mind got stuck on a certain thought or image. Then this thought or image got replayed in your mind over and over again no matter what you did. You don't want these thoughts; it's been said it feels like an avalanche, and along with the thoughts come intense feelings of anxiety. Anxiety is your brain's warning system. When you feel anxious it feels like you are in danger. Also, anxiety is an emotion that tells you to respond, react, protect yourself, and do something. On the one hand, you might recognize that the fear doesn't make sense, doesn't seem reasonable yet it still feels very real, intense, and true. Why would your brain lie? Why would you be experiencing feelings if they weren't true? Feelings don't lie. Unfortunately, if you have OCD, they do lie. If you have OCD, the warning system in your brain is not working correctly.

According to the National Institute of Mental Health (NIMH), your brain is telling you that you are in danger when you are not. When scientists compare pictures of the brains of groups of people with OCD, they can see that on average some areas of the brain are different compared to individuals who don't have OCD. Because of an individual with OCD neurological problems, it is understandable that they are flood with false, scary messages. Further, they buy into these false messages because their warning system (meant to alert them to danger and causing them to panic) is activated falsely.

In addition, people with OCD cannot evaluate OCD thoughts logically, at least without a lot of training says NIMH. One coping technique clinical professional's use to tackle OCD is trying piggybacking reality therapy. Piggybacking reality teaches you to ask yourself how a person without OCD would evaluate a thought. For example, a person with OCD might go over a bump while driving and fear that he has hit someone, causing him to turn around repeatedly to check. To attack this fear, the person can be taught to piggyback. Here is how it works. The person chooses someone without OCD who he/she trusts greatly, and metaphorically, puts that person on his shoulder (similar to symbolic idea of good devil and bad devil). When you experience an OCD thought, the person asks himself how the person on his shoulder would evaluate the situation. The shoulder person likely would say, "If I hit someone, I would know it." Taking it further, the person on the shoulder would say, "If I hit someone I would have heard something, or seen something, and felt something. I certainly would not turn around." Another coping technique clinical professional's use for OCD is called Reality Testing it can be very helpful. Reality testing means asking you how likely is it this will even occur or will not occur.

    Further, it asks what evidence you have for believing this and whether others, who do not have OCD, would interpret your evidence as you do. For example, suppose your jacket brushes by a wall and you notice that there is some dried blood on the wall. Immediately, you worry that you could have contracted AIDS from this blood. Reality testing will have you ask question such as: what is the likelihood that you could contract a disease from your jacket brushing against blood on the wall? How likely is it that the blood contained the AIDS virus? If the blood was dried, how likely is it that a virus could still be transmitted?

"You are not your illness."

--Healthline--

REACTIVE DISTRACTION/PROACTIVE DISTRACTION

It's been said that distractions are good and helps OCD clients. But are they always beneficial when dealing with OCD? I don't think so. Experts believe, distraction, like avoidance, might become a type of compulsion, a way to counteract the anxiety and tear stemming from an obsession. Of course, many well meaning people including some therapists encourage the use of distraction by saying things like, "just think of something else." For example, if you are dealing with a harm obsession, just switch your thoughts to cuddy kittens or puppies (oh, if only it were that easy to "switch our thoughts,") or perhaps distract yourself through an activity, like listening to your favorite music. Try anything to get your mind off the tormenting obsession.

Unfortunately, these distractions will only offer temporary relief (some people will say a temporary relief is better than none), at best, and the obsessions will likely return, stronger than ever. Those who are familiar with Exposure and Response Prevention (ERP) therapy will realize this use of distractions is counter-productive. Research shows what OCD sufferers really need to do is to not distract themselves from the anxiety, but to allow their selves to feel it, in all its intensity. In that way it is a true exposure. So it seems to me there are different types of distraction. Living life to the fullest can provide what some call proactive distractions. Keeping busy takes focus off OCD and allows you to enjoy your life. Don't give OCD any more of your time that you have to. But a distraction that's a direct response to an obsession is what clinical professional's call a reactive distraction. It is similar to a compulsion in that it reduces anxiety in the moment, but ultimately allows OCD to strengthen.

In addition, OCD thoughts are persistent in their determination to get your attention. It is up to you to distract yourself with an activity that is intriguing. It is said, OCD thoughts will not hang around for long unless you give them attention. So, refusing to give attention to your OCD thoughts is essential. And the only way to do this is distraction. Another way is to REVALUE.

Experts believe, revalue is when you tell yourself the messages that cause you so much pain are false, the result of the medical condition are not worth any attention. Research shows, telling yourself that you are going to stab your children or contract AIDS from touching a table has no more validity than telling yourself you are really a rhinoceros. It's been said, watching your OCD morph is also very helpful. People with OCD believe that they are really worried about whatever their current obsession might be. But this is not true. The fact is that once they hold out and give this obsession enough time to pass, another obsession will take its place. Realizing that OCD constantly changes form is helpful because it helps you realize that it is not the particular worry but your neurological condition that has you so upset.

""Tomorrow never comes, it is always today."

--Osho-

VISUALIZATION/GUIDED IMAGERY THERAPY

Guided Imagery Therapy is a traditional mind-body technique that is also considered a form of hypnosis says Dr. Weil. Visualization and guided imagery offer to direct one's concentration on images held in the mind's eye. These therapies take advantage of the connection between the visual brain and the involuntary nervous system. When this portion of the brain (the visual cortex at the back of the head) is activated, without receiving direct input from the eyes, it can influence physical and emotional states says Dr. Weil.

This, in turn, can help elicit physiologic changes in the body, including therapeutic goals. Guided imagery can be learned from books, self-help tapes, CDs, DVDs or in an interactive format utilizing a licensed practitioner to facilitate these techniques, initially, guided imagery involves achieving a state of relaxation. Most clients begin by lying down or sitting in a comfortable chair, loosening any thigh fitting clothes, and disabling common distractions, including televisions, cell phones and computers. After the client gets comfortable, breathing techniques, music, progressive muscle relaxation or a guided induction is often used to help promote a state of deep calm.

In addition, for some people who have never tried guided imagery or hypnosis, the idea of getting deeply relaxed or going into a hypnotic trance may seem frightening. But the fact shows that we've all experienced trance states in everyday life; daydreaming, watching a movie, driving home on autopilot, or practicing meditation or other relaxation techniques. Essentially, trance is simply an altered state of consciousness marked by decreased scope and increased intensity of awareness says Dr. Weil. What distinguishes guided imagery and other forms of hypnosis is that it involves a deliberate choice to enter this state of consciousness for a goal beyond relaxation; to focus your concentration and use suggestion to promote healing. A person in trace is always under control, just as someone who is daydreaming can decide to go on or stop at any time. While a practitioner serves as a teacher or guide, the only person who can allow the shift in consciousness is you, since trance is a latent potential of your own mind.

Therefore, all hypnosis/imagery is self-hypnosis/imagery. It is the self-directed aspect of this therapy that Dr. Weil finds particularly appealing, as he believes that patients do best when they have an understanding and control over the therapies that they use for healing.

> *"Man only likes to count his troubles; he doesn't calculate his happiness."*
>
> *--Flodor Dostoyevsky--*

MEDITATION

Researchers discovered, due to society's wish for a healthier and more natural lifestyle, meditation has been gaining massive popularity as an alternative OCD treatment. Here is why, meditation has been used for centuries to quit, heal, and train the mind. Unlike medication, there aren't any side effects involved. Study has shown, meditation is effective in the treatment of OCD because it removes negative thoughts and feelings, such as stress, guilt, and anxiety, by gaining control of the mind via meditation, impulses, obsessions, and compulsions can no longer control us.

As you might expect, most techniques used for treating OCD involve relaxation and the elimination of "mental noise." Researchers have documented meditation is by far the most effective method of achieving a quite, distraction free, focused mind, quickly disciplining the sufferer to avoid falling back into their compulsive rituals. By providing an environment where threatening ideas are near impossible, meditation effectively makes OCD a thing of the past.

In addition, the practice of self-healing meditation is resting the mind in silence and space, allowing it time to recover and rejuvenate. Mediation does not mean sitting in a perfect state of peace while having no thoughts. Big misconception, the fact show meditation is about establishing a different relationship with your thoughts, just for a little while. Instead of attention being drawn off by whatever thought happens to present itself, in meditation, you watch your thoughts from a different, more stabilized perspective. You're training yourself to place your attention where and when you want. This is very powerful and it gives you the ability to direct your thoughts (mood) in more productive and peaceful directions.

As it been demonstrated in the last few years, this ability has profound self-healing implications for physical and mental health.

> *"Once you're labeled as mentally ill, and that's in your medical notes, then anything you say can be discounted as an artifact of your mental illness."*
>
> --Hilary Mantel--

SELF SOOTHING ACTIVITY

Usually soothing activities are related to the senses. Different people are comforted in different ways and may prefer one sense over another. Sometimes what is soothing for one situation is not the same as what is soothing in a different situation. When your alert system is firing danger, then physical activity may help, like playing a fast moving game of racquetball or going for a walk.

On the other hand, when what is upsetting you is more about feeling hurt or sad, activities such as sipping hot tea or petting a dog may be more effective. Also, the smell of apple pie baking, a beautiful sunset, the softness of a dog's fur, the song of birds singing, the taste of chocolate or the sensation of rocking. Reading a good book can be soothing for some. More examples are being with a good friend, someone you feel safe with and loved by can be soothing.

Another way to be soothed is by focusing on a specific sense. Some people are more visual than others and some are more auditory. Experiment with the different senses to see what works best for you. A self-soothing experience may involve more than one sense and have an overall feel of valuing the self. Having your favorite meal at a table set with cloth napkins and pretty dishes while listening to music with someone you love would be a self-soothing experience for some. Or a bubble bath with your favorite scent, a favorite drink, and listening to a book on tape could also be a self-soothing experience.

Also, in upset moments, it's hard to think about calming yourself. Self-soothing does not come naturally to everyone and requires thoughts and action. Marsha Linehan recognized the importance of self-soothing and included these skills when she developed Dialectical Behavior Therapy. Self-soothing is part of finding a middle ground, a gray area, between being detached or numb and experiencing an emotional crisis or upheaval says Linehan.

She goes on to say hen you allow yourself to experience the uncomfortable emotions (without feeding them and making them more intense) it enables the emotions to pass. Soothing yourself helps you tolerate the experience without acting in ways that are not helpful in the long run, or blocking the emotions, which makes the emotions grow larger or come out in ways you didn't intend. Usually soothing activities are related to the senses.

"Please don't confuse me with my illness, I am not Bipolar, I have bipolar."

--G.E. Laine--

PROS AND CONS FOR OCD

Pros:

- There's almost never a mistake that you've made that you didn't catch and or fix before   it become a full blown disaster.

- You always remember where you last left your car keys.

- Everything you do almost feels like you've looked it away in an emotional Rolodex.

- Important pieces of info like you're driver's license, SS, and passwords to hundreds of things is permanently tattooed into your brain.

- You almost never owe anyone many. Except when you do, and you remember exactly how much. (Word Press)

Cons:
- You're stuck being ridiculous because you're worried that you've left the garage door open when you've already checked it a few times.

- Also, the stove, you think the stove might have been left on.

- You second, guess everything you do because you feel like checking it three times is the magic number.

- You fret over tiny things like where the hell my car keys are if you don't feel them right away in your pocket.

- You have rituals for EVERYTHING. (Word Press)

It's been said, living with obsession and having a name to call it (OCD) is both a blessing and a curse. It's like you could get treatment, but would mean lobotomizing a part of your personality. Can you imagine a day where you are care-free and free from worry ALL THE TIME? It's ironic, I know. "The prison is also a delay to freedom because of precision." (Word Press)

"What lies behind us and what lies before us are tiny matters compared to what lies within us."
--Ralph Waldo Emerson--

OBSERVE YOUR BEHAVIOR

Research shows most people struggling with OCD either view themselves as mad, bad and/or dangerous or they fear that they will become such, so they often go to great lengths to prevent bad things from happening to themselves or to their loved ones. But ask yourself how an observer might judge your values based on your actions. If you spend hours each day trying to protect the people you love, are you really a bad person? If you exert incredible amounts of time and effort to show how much you care, how faithful you are, how you just want others to be safe and happy, maybe you're not so bad or dangerous after all.

And, as for being crazy, there's nothing senseless about OCD. People sometimes fail to understand how rational and logical obsessions and compulsions can be. Remember, your values and behavior is the best reflection of what you are, not those pesky unwanted noisy thoughts, says OCD professionals.

In addition, you can try to create a tape of your OCD obsessions. Experts believe you can focus on one specific worry or obsession and record it to a tape recorder, laptop, or smart phone. Recount the obsessive phrase, sentence, or story exactly as it comes into your mind. Play the tape back to yourself, over and over for a 45-minute period each day, until listening to the obsession no longer causes you to feel highly distressed. Study has shown by continuously confronting your worry or obsession you will gradually become less anxious. You can then repeat the exercise for a different obsession.

Remember to try to be mindful about your OCD, say to yourself that you notice that you are having xyz obsessive thoughts and rate your anxiety out of 10 to yourself. It is said, this technique will help you distance yourself from your OCD without trying to push it away. Also, it's important to remember that no one is perfect, nor can anyone recovery perfectly. Even in well-maintained recoveries, people can occasionally slip up and forget what they are supposed to be doing.

Luckily, there is always another chance to re-expose yourself and so, rather than a person beating yourself up and facing that which is feared, remember no one is perfect. Finally, because health is the result of living in a state of balance, it is extremely important, post-therapy, to live a balanced life, with enough sleep proper diet and exercise, social relationships, and productive work of some type.

"Have patience with all things, but chiefly have patience with yourself. Do not lose courage in considering your own imperfections but instantly set about remedying them-every day begins the task anew."

--Saint Francis de Sales--

Chapter 10

BOUNDARIES AND LIMITS

According to Jacques Lacon, counseling professional, personal boundaries are guidelines, rules or limits that a person creates to identify for them what are reasonable, safe and permissible ways for other people to behave around him or her, and how they will respond when someone steps outside those limits. "They are built out of a mix of beliefs, opinions, attitudes, past experiences and social learning" says Lacon.

Also, physical boundaries provide a barrier between you and intruding force, like a band-aid protects a wound from bacteria. Physical boundaries include your body, sense of person space, and sexual orientation. These boundaries are expressed through clothing, shelter, noise tolerance, verbal instruction, and body language. Other examples of physical boundary invasions are inappropriate touching, such as unwanted sexual advances. Also, looking through others email, phone, and journal is an invasion. It is said, emotional boundaries protect your sense of self-esteem and ability to separate your feelings from others; when you have weak emotional boundaries, it's like getting caught in the midst of a hurricane with no protection and you expose yourself to being greatly affected by others, words, thoughts, and action and end up feeling bruised, wounded, and battered. These include beliefs such as, behaviors, choices, sense of responsibility, and your ability to be intimate with others says Lacon.

According to some in the counseling profession, personal boundaries help to define an individual by outlining likes and dislikes, and setting the distances one allows others to approach. "They include physical, mental, psychological and spiritual boundaries, involving beliefs, emotions, intuitions and self-esteem." "Jacques Lacan considered them to be layered in a hierarchy, reflecting "all the successive envelops of the biological and social status of the person" from the most primitive to the most advance. Personal boundaries operate in two directions, affecting both the incoming and outgoing interactions between people."

In addition, in Nina Brown's self-help book, there are four main types of psychological boundary. One, "a person with soft boundaries merges with other people's boundaries." Someone with a soft boundary is easily a victim of psychological manipulation.

Two, spongy, a person with spongy boundaries is like a combination of having soft and rigid boundaries. They permit less emotional contagion than soft boundaries but more than those with rigid. People with spongy boundaries are unsure of what to let in and what too keep out.

Three, rigid, a person with rigid boundaries is closed or walled off so nobody can get close to him/her either physically or emotionally. "This is often the case if someone has been the victim of physical abuse, emotional abuse, psychological abuse, or sexual abuse." It is said rigid boundaries can be selective which depend on time, place or circumstances and are usually based on a bad previous experience in a similar situation.

Four, flexible, similar to selective rigid boundaries but the person has more control. The person decides what to let in and what to keep out, is resistant to emotional contagion and psychological manipulation, and is difficult to exploit. It's been said individual with mental illness can experience all four types of psychological boundaries.

OPERATE FROM YOUR HEAD (INTELLECTUALLY), HEART (EMOTIONALLY), AND GUT ((INTUITIVELY)

Most of my client's use the expression, follow your "head and not their heart." They go on to suggest when experiencing a mental illness, this is very hard to do. It's been said our head is where the analysis, logic, thoughts and that crazy monkey mind reside. It's also where we think through things, review those "pro's and con's" lists and it's also where fear resides says Rayan Howes, Ph.D, a clinical psychologist, let's consider what some would call the "monkey mind." "The monkey mind thinks of mask fear as "rational thinking."

Experts believe, it comes up with all the reasons to stay in our safe comfort zone and it fears change so it explains why your future change isn't in your best interest. When those fears present themselves, it's time for your True Self to face them and determine how real they are. Until we do that, our fears will control us and greatly limit us.

On the other hand, our heart is where our intuition lies. It is said it's the source of that little voice that guides us, if we let it. Our heart is where our true self resides, our higher self, the one that truly knows what is best for us. Without practice, it's harder to hear our heart and the monkey can take over. The chattering monkey mind speaks so loudly, sending us in different directions without an overall purpose. The monkey makes it hard to hear the heart. When we're busy being busy, the monkey rules. But when we can get quiet, we can finally hear the music in our heart.

In addition, according to some in the counseling professional's, before we make any decisions, from very basic to life-changing, we must learn to pause.

We have to learn to utilize the space between stimulus and responses. During that pause, we need to consider whether the decision we're about to make supports our highest values. Do you know what your highest values are? Most people don't even stop to consider their values because they have no idea what they are. To find out what they are just pick out the three to five most important things to you in life and that's your values. These are the kinds of things that won't change much over a lifetime. My three highest values are my health, my family and my integrity. Each day I practice making choices based on those values. As you think of your own, life, would you say you operate from your head (intellectually), from your heart (emotionally), or from your gut (intuitively)?

It's been said people who make the best decisions typically operate from all three. Your mind, emotions, and intuition should all be cooperating and working together to formulate a reality-based plan that you can operate. Are you someone who chronically gets involved with the wrong person over and over again, never getting your needs met because you operate from your heart and emotions and you don't pay attention to your intellect or your intuition? Did you recognize early on in this relationship that this person was not giving back to you the time, attention or money that you were giving to them? And yet you continue to ignore the signs (intellect) in the hope that there will be payback some day?

"The problem is not that there are problems. The problems is expecting otherwise and thinking that having problems is a problem."

--Theodore L. Rubin--

KEEP YOUR DISTANCE

We may not always be aware of boundary until someone pushes past it triggering feelings of discomfort, anxiety or anger. When these feelings are triggered keep your distance. It can be confusing to feel such strong negative emotions and not be aware of just what triggered them. So it's important when we have such experiences that we ask ourselves if we have discovered something about ourselves; such as is there a boundary here that I wasn't consciously monitoring? What am I learning about myself? Is there anything that I need to do to make sure that this person doesn't cross the boundary again? Setting boundaries and having others honor them is easier said than done especially if you are dealing with mental illness. Just remember not everyone we have relationships with set their boundaries in the same places that we have our own.

In other words, there may be people that you would like to be closer, but the other person keeps you at a distance. Or there may be people that you keep at a distance who want or think that they should be able to be closer. Communication experts feel, an important part of assuming responsibility for teaching people how to treat us is giving a person feedback about the impact of their actions on us. If the act is an error, educate the person. If the act is a violation, remind them that you have talked to them about this before and insist that they honor your personal limits. Often these are difficult conversations.

However, it's a conversation that you are entitled to have for the benefit of your own safety, integrity, and health. According to some in the counseling profession, here are some skills you should know that will help you set boundaries in your life. You must first learn to communicate without blaming. In other words, stop saying things like; you make me so angry; you hurt me; you make me crazy; how could you do that to me after all I have done for you; etc. these are the very types of messages we got in childhood that have so warped our perspective on our own emotional process. Instead use "I statements". "I feel frustrated or angry when…..or when xyz happens". Also, along with good communication you need honesty. Learn to say how you feel because beating around the bush will not help you or your relationship in the long run and will be easier for you to share your mental illness if needed. It is impossible to set boundaries without setting consequences. If you are setting boundaries in a relationship, and you are not yet at point where you are ready to leave the relationship then don't say that you will leave.

    Lastly, never state something that you are not willing to follow through with says Indiana University, Purdue University on boundaries.

"I think Hell exists on Earth. It's a psychological state, or it can be a physical state. People who have severe mental illness are in Hell. People who have lost a loved one are in Hell. I think there are all kinds of different hells. It's not a place you go to after you die."

--Al Franken--

SAYING NO

How many times have you said "yes," "sure," or "no problem" to a request only to immediately regret you response? You may find yourself committed to giving your time, effort, money or energy to something you have little or no desire to participate in.

Often, we are caught off guard or obligated with various requests from people well intended and we feel the urge to immediately say yes in compliance. This only leads to anguish, remorse and stress. It is said each time you agree when you don't want to, you give up a piece of yourself. This can lead to feelings of powerlessness because you are in another person's grip, fulfilling her/his wishes or meeting his/her needs and not your own. Saying no is a learned skill. If you are a master of yes and a learner of no, the process of learning how to change can seem distressing and cause anxiety. While saying no probably won't change your personality, it will help you assert yourself. It's been suggested it could even put an end to that empty feeling in the pit of your stomach when you commit beyond your stamina or to the point of draining your emotional nerves. A calmer life, under your own supervision, will be the outcome.

To add, communication experts suggested these five steps to help you learn to say NO. First, make a list, just as you would track spending for budget purposes, track how many times you say yes during any give week. Being aware of the habit of people pleasing is the first step in making desired changes for personal empowerment. Two, know how you are spending your time; once you know how often you agree with others, it will become clear how you are spending your time. It will help you find out if one particular person or activity monopolizing the majority of your time? Three, get your priorities straight; if you don't know what is important to you what you value most how can you possibly choose when to say yes and when to say no? Four, your values, beliefs and priorities should be demonstrated in your actions and your choices. Five, give some control to others; many times we agree to take on more than we can because we enjoy being in control.

Or, we may feel someone else cannot complete a given project as well. When you are able to trust other people you will feel the ease in giving over some control identify your boundaries; a boundary is a limit on how far you can go with comfort, both emotionally and physical. A boundary is also present and a clear limit. It is personal and is set by you.

> "The true definition of mental illness is when the majority of your time is spent in the past or future, but rarely living in the realism of NOW."
>
> --Shannor L. Alder--

BE FIRM

If you're uncomfortable being so firm, or are dealing with pushy people, it's ok to say, "Let me think about it and get back to you." This gives you a chance to review your schedule, as well as your feelings about saying "yes" to another commitment, do a cost-benefit analysis, and then get back to them with a yes or no says communication experts. Most importantly, this tactic helps you avoid letting yourself be pressured into over scheduling your life and taking on too much stress.

According to some in the counseling professional's, being firm not defensive or overly apologetic and polite gives the signal that you are sympathetic, but will not easily change your mind if pressured. If you decide to tell the person you'll get back to them, be mater-of-fact and not too promising. If you lead people to believe you'll likely say "yes" later, they'll be more disappointed with a later "no." Be firm, but nice. Experts believe believes one of the reasons you may hesitate to say no is because you think it will make you look "bitchy" or selfish, but that can be avoided by finding a pleasant way to say it. Rather than saying abruptly, "no", I won't help you with this," you could say apologetically. "I'm really sorry, but I just can't do it at this time and maybe another time. The majority of people will understand and will not be upset.

However, if you do receive resistance, that is the time to become more firm in your answers. One of the hardest parts of setting boundaries is learning to be firm with you. You may be tempted to overextend yourself to help others, even when you know it wouldn't be in your best interests. When that temptation arises, you'll have to be able to override your desire to please and do what you know is best for yourself.

In addition, it's been said being firm without being rude can be thought of as being an art in itself. The assertive person is someone who is a master of this art. According to some in the counseling profession, one technique for being firm without being rude is what is said to be called the "mirror effect." Most people hate it when a person mimics their actions and words, but this technique can be used to give people a dose of their own medicine.

For example, let's say you work in an office next to someone, and you one day notice that they are leaving traces of trash near your cubicle. You are naturally irritated by this, and you have the option of confronting the person about it in a hostile way. Aggressive people would do this, while passive people would ignore the situation or put the trash in the trash can without saying anything. In contrast, someone who uses the mirror effect would begin leaving trash in the other person's cubicle area. If this person complains about it, you can respond by calmly saying that you were just showing them what it is like to have trash in their cubicle area, since they have been doing the same to you. In most cases, the person will get it, especially if you are calm about it. As the famous Spanish writer Baltasar Gracian said, "The truth of seen, rarely heard". If you can show people that you are firm without being aggressive, then you will become a master of not only your personal relationships, but your business relationships as well says the counseling profession.

"It is in my head! That's why it's called Mental Illness."
--Roni Askey Doran--

BE ASSERTIVE

It's been said assertiveness is a very important means for communicating your needs in a way that is fair to both yourself and to others. Unfortunately, for some insecure people, assertive people are sometimes threatening and it is easier to label them as arrogant, selfish, or unhelpful when they receive the answer "no" or when boundaries are made clear by the assertive person. In particular, those with manipulation, neediness, and trust problems can see assertive responses as undermining their own agendas and will seek to respond with negative critiques of an assertive person's behavior. This is where it can get a little tricky for the newly assertive convert but it's no reason to suddenly start worrying that you are arrogant!

It is said, to be assertive is to assert or express your rights, to stand up for yourself and your values and beliefs, and to be able to express your true feelings openly. It is to be able to declare yourself, who you are, what you think and feel. It is an active rather than a passive approach to others, and to life.

Also, experts believe, assertiveness in communication and social relationships involves openness, honesty, and firmness, all with appropriateness and flexibility. The assertive person is confident in a relaxed way, as well as free and spontaneous in social situations. Human being has a right, and even a responsibility, to assert their rights. Studies has shown, to do otherwise is to go around half alive, passive, inhibited, cowed and submitting, even suffering such complaints as headaches, stomach disturbances, general fatigue, rashes, and so on.

In addition, non-assertive individuals seldom feel happy with or proud of themselves; in fact, they often put themselves down in a rather destructive way. On the other hand, when assertiveness goes too far and takes advantage of others, it is aggression. Aggressive behavior cuts across the rights of others, attacks them and puts them down; it is destructive, hurts people and makes them feel badly. Aggressive individuals may feel on top of things, but they will be watching in case someone tries to better them. They are often defensive, and seldom have many friends says University of Victoria Counseling Services.

"The healing process is best described as a spiral. Survivors go through the stages once, sometimes many times; sometimes in one order, sometimes in another. Each time they hit a stage again, they move up the spiral; they can integrate new information and a broader range of feelings, utilize more resources, take better care of themselves, and make deeper changes."

--Laura Hough--

BE SPECIFIC

When someone has crossed your boundary, share a specific, detailed response. According to Hanks, Student Affairs Counseling Center, rather than saying "You're so controlling," say: "When I gave my feedback in the meeting yesterday, it seem like you quickly dismissed it without consideration. That hurt and I don't like it. Will you be aware of that next time? I'd like at least a few minutes to share my ideas with the team. When someone has crossed your boundary, share a specific, detail response. Boundaries are keys for your well-being and your relationships. In fact, they're essential "if you want to live a life you love says Black, Student Affairs Counseling Center. When we take ourselves and our priorities seriously, others will, too, she said, "boundaries show we are serious about living our lives in ways we believe are best for us." "The people around us will adjust to them or leave. "Bless them either way."

In addition, as I previously stated, using "I" statement is the key to good communication. Using vague or tentative statements will likely lead to misinterpretation. The following statements project this preciseness: "I feel…", "I don't want to…." "I have mixed reactions. I agree with these aspects for these reasons, but I'm distressed about these aspects for these reasons." Acknowledge that your message comes from your frame of reference and your perceptions. You can acknowledge ownership with personalized ("I) statements such as "I don't agree with you" (as compared to "You're wrong"). Ask for feedback and then listen carefully to the other person. "Am I being clear?" Does that make sense? How do you see this situation? What do you want to do? Asking for feedback can make it clear to the other person that you are expressing an opinion, feeling, or desire rather than a demand.

Listening to their feedback and engaging in a discussion can correct any misperceptions either of you have. Encourage others to be clear, direct, and specific in their feedback to you. Remember it takes time, support, and relearning to be able to set effective boundaries. Self-awareness and learning to be assertive are the first steps. Setting boundaries isn't selfish. Its self-love, you say, "yes" to yourself each time you say "no." It builds self-esteem. But it usually takes encouragement to make yourself a priority and to persist, especially when you receive pushback. Read more on setting boundaries in codependency for dummies.

"Once a restless or frayed mood has turned to anger, or violence, or psychosis, Richard, like most, finds it very difficult to see it as illness, rather than being willful, angry, irrational or simply tiresome."

--Kay Redfield Jamison--

DON'T BE A DOORMAT

You know what they say, if you act like a doormat, people will walk all over you...so don't to be afraid to say NO. Don't be afraid to say what YOU WANT; don't be afraid to say that is NOT acceptable, or you CANNOT talk to me that way, you CANNOT treat me that way. Don't be afraid to let them walk out of your life because you don't need them. It is you responsibility when they continue to mistreat you to draw a line in the sand and either walk away or do something about it because you cannot blame someone else for treating you badly when you let them. Are you being treated like a doormat? Are you sick and tired of people walking all over you? Are you ready to change your situation..? Being a doormat to someone you care about is a very hard situation to be in and to get yourself out of. You have to realize that you as an individual person deserve respect and to not be talked down to all the time. It might be you don't believe in yourself enough or not worthy so you're stuck believing you're not good enough or worthy enough. You aren't enough or you don't do enough. It's been said if you were taught to always value someone else's opinion more than your own, you probably will always be in search of someone's approval. So it's easier to please everyone and be a doormat. I realize this is difficult subject for some.

In addition, no one wants to be a doormat. But if we're not careful, we can easily end up feeling used up and stepped on. How do you define someone who is a doormat? A doormat is simply a person who allows people to treat them badly or walk all over them. Do you allow people to take advantage of you and you never speak up? Is it so difficult to say "no" to someone, when you would prefer to do so? Do you avoid speaking your mind; or rarely state your opinion in case it's different from the group; you avoid getting angry; you change your opinion to fit in. You tend to be attracted to 'controlling' people.

It's been said setting boundaries can make an enormous impact on the quality of your life. It is a major step in taking control of your life and quality of your life and vital for taking responsibility for yourself and your life. It is the one skill that you need the most to develop in order to create the kind of life you really want. However, it's often the area where most people seem to have most difficulties. We know that sometimes in life people (try to) walk all over you for no apparent reason and despite your good intentions, they just run rough-shade over you, doing whatever they want in the way they want, as long as they get what they want. If this is happening to you then you might be a doormat. If you try to be who someone else wants you to be. Apologize a lot or afraid to rock the boats then you're a doormat.

Also, if you often say "yes" when you want to say" No"; you avoid speaking your mind. Or rarely state your opinion in case it's different from the group; you avoid getting angry; you change your opinion to fit in. Also, doormats tend to be attracted to 'controlling' people.

"We have a mental health system that is dominated by political and hidden forces that keep us stagnated and unable to see real, lasting change."

--Tamara Hill--

BODY LANGUAGE

Body language technically known as kinesics is a significant aspect of modern communications and relationships. It's been said Body language is very relevant to management and leadership, and to all aspects of work and business where communications can be seen and physically observed among people. Body language is also very relevant to relationships outside of work, for example in dating and mating, and in families and parenting. Listening is a big part of communication. In terms of observable body language, non-verbal signals are being exchanged whether these signals are accompanied by spoken words or not. Body language goes both ways; your own body language reveals your feelings and meanings to others or other people's body language reveals their feelings and meanings to you. The sending and receiving of body language signals happens on conscious and unconscious levels. Appropriate body language is an important aspect of assertive behavior. Good posture and eye contact are a must. Slouching is said it signals that you are unsure of yourself. Refusing to maintain enough eye contact suggests that you are untrustworthy. Staring into someone's eyes and refusing to look away is just as bad. It makes people uncomfortable and is a sign of aggressive, not assertive, behavior.

In addition, by becoming more aware of this body language and understanding what it might mean, you can learn to read people more easily. This puts you in a better position to communicate effectively with them. Also, by increasing your understanding of others, you can also become more aware of the messages that you convey to them. There are times when we send mixed messages; we say one thing yet out body language reveals something different. This non-verbal language will affect how we act and react to others, and how they react to us. As you observe others, you can identify some common signs and signals that give away whether they are feeling confident or not. Typical things to look for in confident people include: posture, standing tall with shoulders back. Eye contact, solid with a smiling face; Gestures with hands arms, purposeful and deliberate, speech, slow and clear, tone of voice, moderate to low. As well as deciphering other people's body language, you can use this knowledge to convey feelings that you're not actually experiencing.

For example, if you are about to enter into a situation where you are not as confident as you'd like to be, such as giving a big presentation or attending an important meeting, you can adopt these confidence signs and signals to project confidence.

"The vision I see in the mirror is me, who I am, supposedly, but that vision does not express the way my mind works or the way I feel inside. A realization creeps over me, the words tumbling into my head quietly like falling leaves."

--Victoria Sawyer--

Chapter 11

ASSERTIVENESS

According to the counseling professionals, assertiveness means standing up for your personal rights, expressing thoughts, feelings and beliefs in direct, honest and appropriate ways. It is important to remember by being assertive we should always respect the thoughts, feelings and beliefs of other people. It is said, assertiveness is to being able to express feelings, wishes, want and desires appropriately and is an important personal and interpersonal skill.

Also, assertiveness in your interactions with other people can help you to express yourself in a clear way without undermining the rights of yourself or others. The facts show, assertiveness is different from aggressiveness; it enables an individual to act in their own best interests, to stand up for themselves without undue anxiety. In addition, assertiveness helps to express honest feelings comfortably and to express personal rights without denying the rights of others. Like most individuals with mental illness, you struggle to be assertive; you are more likely to crumble than stand up for yourself. You may also find it hard to tell people what you want in any given situation, whether it's with colleagues, dealing with pushy friends or a distracted partner who seems more interested in the football results than your request to clean up what use to be called a kitchen.

Experts believe, a lack of assertiveness is inextricably linked with a lack of confidence and low self-esteem, chronic stress, depression, anxiety disorders, anger issues, relationship and parenting problems, workplace bullying the list goes on. In other words, if you don't feel good about yourself, deep down, it's hard to ask for what you need.

Overcoming this may not be easy, but the good news is a few simple techniques that you will learn throughout this chapter can help you become more assertive.

To start, let's look at how assertiveness is defined. It will help if you think about the three different states passivity, aggression and assertiveness. It's been said when you are passive, we tend to speak quietly and make ourselves physically small; we will let others take the lead and avoid making decisions, often for fear of criticism or rejection. Whereas, when we are aggressive, we're at the other end of the spectrum, speaking loudly and being dominant; we may bully others into doing what we want, either verbally or physically; we may well be prone to angry outburst which, although they feel powerful at the time, are destructive and ultimately disempowering, because we have to deal with the consequences.

On the other hand, assertiveness is a state in which we calmly and clearly express our thoughts and feelings; our body posture is open and upright, our gestures expressive; we make eye contact with the other person and listen carefully to what they have to say before replying. Although we ask for what we want and try to get our needs met, we don't do so at any cost if necessary, we seek a compromise so it's a win-win, not an "I win-you lose" situation.

AGGRESSIVE

When you respond in an aggressive way, the rights and self-esteem of the other person are undermined. Counseling professionals suggested aggressive responses can include a wide range of behaviors, like rushing someone unnecessarily, telling rather than asking, ignoring someone, or not considering another's feelings. Also, aggressive behavior fails to consider the views or feelings of other individuals and it rarely will praise or allow appreciation of others be shown, and an aggressive response tends to put others down.

According to research documents, aggressive responses encourage the other person to respond in a non-assertive way, either aggressively or passively. It can be a frightening or distressing experience to be spoken to aggressively and the receiver can be left wondering what instigated such behavior or what he or she has done to deserve the aggression. When thoughts and feelings are not stated clearly, this can lead to individuals manipulating others into meeting their wishes and desires. Manipulation can be seen as a cover form of aggression at the same time humor can also be used aggressively.

According to Brian Murray, MS, "Feeling Angry," it may sound contradictory for an angry person to be more assertive, however being more assertive can help release built up anger. Anger is a normal emotion and we all experience it at one time or another. However, there are times when we have a tendency to hold things in regarding issues in life such as a perceived injustice or the lack of boundaries. When anger goes unexpressed for too long it can turn inward manifesting into resentment and compulsive behaviors says Murry. It is not uncommon for anger held on to for long periods of time to turn into depression. As has been mentioned, other symptoms of mismanaged anger can be strong just of sarcasm, isolation, substance abuse, relationship problems and a general sense of the loss of self. Anger manifested outward is much more obvious. It can appear as directed at inanimate objects, road rage, yelling or becoming abusive toward others. In other words, you can avoid some of these symptoms by just learning how to be assertive properly.

Lastly, as has been mentioned, it's important to be assertive to avoid experiencing; depression, anger turned inward, a sense of being helpless, hopeless, or of having no control over your life. Also, you can avoid feeling resentful to others for manipulating or taking advantage of you or feeling frustration, such as asking, why did I allow that to happen? Additionally, you can create temper/violence, if you can't express anger appropriately, it may build up. Most people find it easier to be assertive in some situations than in others. This makes perfect sense. It's a lot easier to hold your ground with a stranger than with someone you love who might get angry if you express your true feelings. But, the more important the relationship to you, the more important it is to be assertive.

"I've got to that point in life when there are very few thrills and lots of pills seem we all end up this way. As we wait for our final day. But there's one thing about the pills I take. My manic episodes have taken a break."

--Stanly Victor Paskavich--

STAY CALM CONFIDENT AND BOOST SELF-ESTEEM

Being assertive is a core communication skill. As has been noted, being assertive means that you express yourself effectively and stand up for your point of view, while also respecting the rights and beliefs of others. Being assertive can also help boost your self-esteem and earn others respect. This can help with stress management as well, especially if you tend to take on too many responsibilities because you have a hard time saying no. Some people seem to be naturally assertive but if you're not one of them, you can learn to be more assertive. Assertiveness is simply based on mutual respect; it's been said it's an effective and diplomatic communication style.

Also, being assertive shows that you respect yourself because you're willing to stand up for your interests and express your thoughts and feelings. And, it demonstrates that you're aware of the right of others and are willing to work on resolving conflicts. It is difficult to maintain all the other aspects of assertive behavior if you are unable to stay calm. So, if you feel yourself losing control and do not think you'll be able to regain it quickly, tell the person with whom you are talking with that you want to take some time to consider what's been said. Then suggest a specific time to resume the discussion.

In addition, counseling professionals suggest the first step we must take is to boost and strengthen our self-esteem and confidence. Think about it, if your self-esteem and confidence with you is low, it will undermine us at every turn. Not having that self-esteem will distract and subtract from our goals, and will inhibit us. Things turn against us because we let it happen through something call self-talk and the wrong kind of self-talk (which a lot of people with mental illness have) only serves to undermine us. So we must combat the self-talk that produces negative comments and situations, and change it. We must make it clear to ourselves about what we want; it's amazing how many things we think we want but don't want. It's surprising how we talk ourselves out of the prize or be allowed to give up the prize or issue at hand, all because we don't want that thing enough or our self-esteem is stopping us. This clarity is vital so that we can counter-act that so-called pep talk or spin or threat we usually get from aggressive people. We get it in the shopping mall, on the doorstep, and conned into buying that thing we never really need anyway. So we must be clear about what we want. We need to know our own value, and believe that we have the very same entitlements and rights as others in order to have our beliefs, our interests and our views respected. This is a hard thing for some people, while easy for others.

"Violet is the most soothing, tranquilizing and cooling color vibration. It encourages the healing of unbalanced mental conditions in people who are overly nervous or high-strung. Foods of the violet vibration are; purple broccoli, beetroot and purple grapes."

--Tae Yun Kim--

BE CONCISE AND TO THE POINT

According to the Oxford Learning Institute of University of Oxford, being assertive takes time and practice and it is a way of behaving that requires effort too. Preparation and practice is the key to success for anything. Spending time thinking about what you are going to say and how you are going to say it will help to ensure your conversation is as effective as possible. You might like to make a few notes, or bullet points before you speak to someone because anyone can forget. You might like to take those notes in with you and refer to them if needed. You do not need to write a script, but a few key points can be helpful. Practicing what you are going to say, out loud is also highly recommended. Over time, demonstrating assertive behavior has also shown to increase self-confidence and self-esteem. Oxford Leaning Institute suggested using these 6 steps to ensure you will have effective conversations with people.

First, plan the outcome, knowing what you want to gain from a situation is vital because if you are not clear in your own mind, you won't have a clear message to express to others. Also, identify your ideal outcome first before deciding on the verbal steps towards attaining it.

Second, be specific and concise, say exactly what you mean and get to the point right away. 'Don't side-track, hint or apologize.

Third, acknowledge what others say and show others that you're genuinely listening to them through responsive body language and by referring back to what they've said. Don't patronize or sympathies, because it disembowel others.

Fourth, show repetition because in order to be heard you might want to repeat your statement two or three times. Do so calmly, clearly, politely, in a steady voice that shows neither irritation nor impatience. This "broken record" technique ensures that your viewpoint is heard.

Fifth, self-disclosure is saying how you feel and taking responsibility for those feelings, specifically by saying "I statements." For example "I feel..." "I think..." "I would like" etc. Or 'I feel concerned about asking you when I know how busy you are at this time of year...' to express how you feel about asserting yourself. Example: 'I felt disappointed that I wasn't consulted about the move as it affects me considerably...' to say how you feel as a consequence of someone's behavior.

Six, a workable compromise, (when appropriate/relevant) in the event that your request isn't granted or you disagree with the other party, seek to find an alternative solution which is acceptable to both parties. Be absolutely clear about what you want. Be direct and specific. State what you want. If there is a problem, state what you think is the problem and what you think will be the best resolution. Do not give anyone the opportunity to misinterpret what you are saying. A good way to make sure that you are being understood is to ask for feedback. Make certain that the person with whom you're speaking knows what you're saying says Oxford Learning Institution.

"Many so-called disorders of the mind are simply disorders of thought."

--Vironika Tugaleva--

ASSERTIVE COMMUNICATION

Communication experts agree the most productive and most effective way to communicate is honestly and openly, which is assertive communication. This type of communication allows the potential for people to also communicate openly and honestly with you. Assertive communication is defined as clear, direct, honest statement of feelings; us of "I" messages; speaking up appropriately for oneself while considering the needs, wants, and right of others.

There is a new study from Stanford Graduate School of Business suggest part of the problem is the lack of confidence to use "I" statements in assertive communication. Here are some tips and guidelines that is suggested to build your assertive communication skills: Visualize the person you want to be. How would that person behave and communicate: Do you currently exhibit this behavior and what do you have to change? Ask for feedback from trusted colleagues about the way you are coming across. This would be a great discussion with a mentor as well. Practice Using "I" statements. Stay true to your feelings without blaming others. State your opinions clearly. Accept compliments with grace. Say "thank you." It's simple but somehow we always find the need to give credit to others or discredit the compliment. Don't downplay the compliment. Take credit.

In addition, practice giving your opinion at least once. Make it a goal to speak when you get the opportunity. Practice saying "no" especially when people delegate inappropriately to you. Ask for what you need. Remember, no one knows everything so acknowledge this. Practice expressing your opinion clearly and confronting issues head-on using "I" statements. Avoid the inclination to backpedal and negate your true feelings.

Build your self-confidence and stay focused on your value. This gives you the courage to communicate effectively. Make sure you are balancing you communication style so that it is not aggressive or passive aggressive. Focus on unhooking emotionally from situations with difficult bosses and colleagues. Instead focus on your reaction. You can't control their behavior. You can only control your reaction. Most of all, being assertive means knowing where the fine line is between assertion and aggression and balancing it. It means having a strong sense of yourself and acknowledging that you deserve to get what you want. And it means standing up for you even in the most difficult situations. Assertiveness can be learned and developed.

Although it won't happen overnight, by practicing the techniques presented here you will slowly become more confident in expressing your needs and wants says Stanford Graduate School of Business. As your assertiveness improves, so will your productivity and efficiency. Start today and begin to see how being assertive allows you to work with people to accomplish tasks, solve problems and reach solutions.

"The presuming social view that mental health is not as serious as the media says it is, blocks progress. This too is political."
--Tamara Hill--

4 IDEAS TO ASSERTIVENESS

According to Paterson, these are 4 ideas to get you started on the road to assertiveness.

1. Start small. You wouldn't try to scale a mountain before reading a manual, practicing on a rock wall and then moving on to bigger peaks. Going in unprepared just sets you up for failure. Paterson suggested trying to be assertive in mildly tense situations, such as requesting to be seated at a different spot at a restaurant. Then gently work up to tougher situations such as talking to your spouse about infidelity issues, he said.

2. Learn to say no. People worry that saying no is selfish. It's not. Rather, setting healthy limits is important to having healthy relationships.

3. Let go of guilt. Being assertive can be tough — especially if you've been passive or a people pleaser most of your life. The first few times it can feel unnerving. But remember that being assertive is vital to your well-being. "Assertive behavior that involves advocating for oneself in a way that is respectful of others is not wrong — it is healthy self-care," Marter said. Sometimes, you might be unwittingly perpetuating your guilty feelings with negative thoughts or worries. "Replace negative thoughts — such as 'I am a bad person for not loaning my friend money' — with a positive mantra [such as] 'I deserve to have financial stability and not put myself in jeopardy,'" she said.

4. Express your needs and feelings. Don't assume that someone will automatically know what you need. You have to tell them. Again, be specific, clear, honest and respectful, Marter said.

For example, ordering food at a restaurant, she said. You'd never just order a "sandwich." Instead you'd request a "tuna on rye with slices of cheddar cheese and tomatoes." If you're worried of upsetting someone, use "I" statements, which usually make people less defensive.

According to Marter, instead of saying, "You have no clue what my life is like, and you are a selfish ass," you might say, "I am exhausted and I need more help with the kids." What also helps is tempering your anger and speaking from a place of hurt, she said, such as: "I feel so lonely and need you to spend time with me."

"Focus on the real issue, not the minutiae," she said. In other words, "are you really mad that the toilet seat was left up or that you were up with the baby five times the night before?" If it's the baby — and it likely is — be clear and specific: "I am upset that I was up with the baby five times last night and need for you to get up at least twice a night."

"My worst days in recovery are better than the best days in relapse."

--Kate Le Page--

Chapter 12

SUICIDAL IDEATION

If you or someone you know is considering suicide and are unsure how to deal with it, call suicide hotline (1-800-SUICIDE) to get help. Researchers have documented, suicidal thoughts are troubling, especially when accompanied by depression, other mental illnesses, alcohol or substance abuse, or plans for suicide. This situation demands immediate evaluation. These thoughts may indicate you have a serious psychological disorder.

Doctor's has said, there is a critical distinction between a person's thoughts regarding death and suicide and actually feeling suicidal. When doctors hear that someone wants to die, they refer to these thoughts as suicidal ideation and divide them into two categories active and passive. It's been said suicidal ideation can be active and involve a current desire and plan to die or a suicidal ideation can also be passive, involving a desire to die but without a plan to bring about one's death. If a person has an actual desire to die (in either form of suicidal ideation), he or she must seek immediate medical attention. The differences between a symptom and a sign are, symptom is something the person senses and describes, while a sign is something other people, such as the doctor notice.

For example, drowsiness may be a symptom while dilated pupils may be a sign. Experts believe the person can appear to feel trapped or hopeless, appearing to have an abnormal preoccupation with violence, dying and/or death. Other examples are they could be in a heightened state of anxiety; be very moody; changing personality; changing routine; changing sleeping patterns; consuming drugs; consuming more alcohol; engaging in risky behavior, such a driving carelessly or taking drugs; getting affairs in order; getting hold of a gun, medications, or substances that could end their life; giving stuff away; having depression; having panic attacks; impaired concentration; increased self-criticism; isolating oneself; psychomotor agitation, such as pacing around a room, wringing one's hand, taking off clothing and putting it back on, and other such actions; saying goodbye to others as if it were the last time; seeming to be unable to experience pleasurable emotions from normally pleasurable life events such as eating, exercise, social interaction or sex; seeming to have severe remorse; talking about killing oneself, expressing regret about being alive or even having been born.

Research shows a significant number of people with suicidal ideation keep their thoughts and feelings a secret and appear to have no apparent signs.

CALL SOMEONE (SUPPORT HOTLINE)

If you have a friend or family member that need your support don't be afraid to ask, start by telling the person you are concerned and give him/her examples. If he/she is depressed, don't be afraid to ask whether he/she is considering suicide, or if he/she has a particular plan or method in mind.

Also, ask if they have a therapist and/or are taking medication. Talking to a friend or family member about their suicidal thoughts and feelings can be extremely difficult for anyone. But if you're unsure whether someone is suicidal, the best way to find out is to ask. You can't make a person suicidal by showing that you care, and no matter what problems they are dealing with, you just want to help them find a reason to keep living. When you call a hotline, (1-800-273-TALK /8255) you'll be connected to a skilled, trained counselor at a crisis center in your area, anytime 24/7. When you dial 1-800-TALK, you are calling the crisis center in the Lifeline network closet to your location. After you call, you will hear a message saying you have reached the National Suicide Prevention Lifeline. You will hear hold music while your call is being routed. You will be helped by a skilled, trained crisis worker who will listen to your problems and will tell you about mental health services in your area. Don't worry your call is confidential and free.

In addition, experts believe the first step to coping with suicidal thoughts and feelings is to share them with someone we trust. It may be a friend, a therapist, a member of the clergy, a teacher, a family doctor, a coach, or an experience counselor at the end of a helpline. The idea is to find someone you trust and let them know how bad things are. Don't let fear, shame, or embarrassment prevent you from seeking help. Just talking about how you got to this point in your life can release a lot of the pressure that's building up and help you find a way to cope. Remember, you're not alone; it's been said many of us have had suicidal thoughts at some point in our lives. Feeling suicidal is not a character defect, and it doesn't mean that you are crazy, or weak, or flawed. It only means that you have more pain that you can cope with right now. This pain seems overwhelming and permanent at the moment, but with time and support, you can overcome your problems and the pain and suicidal feelings wills pass. It's been suggested by professional's to join a support group.

In addition, many organizations around the country run support groups for people with different types of mental health problems. One of the great benefits about support groups are, you can link with some group members and can support each other and learn from each other's ways of coping. You can call the Mind Info-line at 300 -123 -3393) for support in your area. Or another option is calling a help lines. If you believe that family and friends don't understand you or that you cannot keep bothering them (especially in the middle of the night) it can be a good idea to phone a helpline, such as Samaritans or PAPYRUS and listen to other people who have suicidal feelings. Keep the number handy so that you aren't hunting around for it in a crisis. You can usually write, email or text if you don't want to talk on the phone. If you do call, the person listening to you will give you the time and space to talk in confidence without judging you. They will not tell you what to do; they will help you think through what to do for yourself.

"I am not what happened to me, I am what I choose t become."
--Carl Jung--

http://therapist2013.wix.com/e-therapy

DON'T ENTERTAIN THE THOUGHTS

Professional counselors suggest not becoming preoccupied with suicidal thoughts because this can make them even stronger. Don't think and rethink negative thoughts find a distraction or think positive. Distraction will give you a break from suicidal thoughts it can help, even if it's for a short period of time. The Mayo Clinic warns that people who may be about to commit suicide will openly talk about it, perhaps as directly as stating, "I am going to kill myself." Because we glibly use language in modern society, it's easy to assume such talk may be a turn of phrase rather than a genuine suicide threat. Psychiatrists tend to agree that the more slight statements about ending one's life are likely serious. Be alert to comments such as, "I wish I had never been born," and "I'd rather be dead."

In addition, there is probably no way that a depressed person at risk of contemplating or attempting suicide can be sufficiently objective to analyze their own situation. If you are experiencing dark thoughts and engage in precise suicide planning, and are able to visualize clearly a world without you in it get professional help immediately. Don't second-guess whether or not you might actually go through with it, get help now. Remember many people think of suicide from time to time. The philosopher Camus noted, "There is but one truly serious philosophical problem and that is suicide."

The philosopher Nietzsche said, "the thought of suicide is great consolation: by means of it one gets through many a dark night." To seriously consider suicide is a sign that something is wrong. Our natural instinct in life is to survive. People endure unimaginable horrors in order to stay alive, as but one example, just think of the man who cut his arm off with a pocket knife in order to liberate his body from a boulder, having been trapped beneath it for five days and seven hours.

If your instinct to survive has become weakened, it is a sign that you need help. Please seek that help, whether from a trusted friend or family member, clergy, physician, therapist, or some other supports you have.

"Prejudices, it is well known, are most difficult to eradicate from the heart whose soil has never been loosened or fertilized by education; they grow there, firm as weeds among stones."
--Charlotte Bronte--

DISTRACTION

One way to become distracted from suicidal thoughts is develop new activities and interests. Find new hobbies, volunteer activities, or work that gives you a sense of meaning and purpose. When you're doing things you find fulfilling, you'll feel better about yourself and feelings of despair are less likely to return. To help you, here are lists of other distractions you can use. Try thinking about what have help you in the past, and write it down.

For example, eating at your favorite restaurant, calling an old friend to talk, watching your favorite TV shows and movies, rereading a favorite book that soothe you, going on a road trip, looking at old emails that make you feel good, hanging out with your dog in the park, going for a long walk or run to clear your head. Studies has shown sometimes coping with your suicidal feelings is simply a matter of waiting until the medication kicks in or your circumstances change. While you are waiting, however, it can help you to find ways to distract yourself from the emotional pain. Make an agreement with yourself that just for a little while (as long as it takes to watch a movie, phone a friend or maybe go to work), you will not focus on your darker thoughts. As you string together these shorter periods of distraction, enough time will eventually pass for you to start feeling better.

In addition, other ideas for distractions are, you can make a distraction box by filling a box with memories and items that can provide comfort and help lift your mood when you feel down. The box can contain anything that is meaningful and helpful to you, such as a CD you like listening to, a book, photos, letters, poems, notes to yourself, a cuddly toy, a perfume, jokes etc. Give yourself a break and take a break from yourself.

If your attention is focused mainly on your misery, try instead to notice the world around you. Just like any new habit, it may take effort at first, especially if you feel cut off and disconnected. Try being kind to your body and exercise regularly like walking, running and swimming, it can lift your spirits and make it easier for you to sleep better. Another is Yoga.

As I mention, yoga and meditation can energies you and help to reduce tension, and a healthy diet can help you feel stronger and may help you feel better. And when you start to feel better, it might help if you put together a list of meals that are easy to prepare. Also, if you have misused alcohol and drugs, cutting down on these will make your mind clearer and better able to focus on how you should help yourself. You might like to write down your thoughts, feelings and achievements (however small) in a daily diary. Or creating artworks based on your feelings can also be a powerful tool. It's been said over time, this can help you see what you are thinking and feeling and can make it easier for you to find ways to respond differently to your difficulties.

"It's a bit like walking down a long, dark corridor never knowing when the light will go on."

--Neil Lennon--

GO TO A PLACE WHERE YOU DO FEEL SAFE

If you are having suicidal thoughts and don't feel safe staying by yourself at home, go to a place where you do feel safe, like a friends' house, your parent's house, or a community center or other public place. It is evidence showing you should identify triggers or situations that lead to feelings of despair or generate suicidal thoughts, such as an anniversary of a loss, alcohol, or stress form relationships. Also, find ways to avoid these places, people or situations. Even if your suicidal thoughts and feelings have subsided, get help for yourself. Experts believe experiencing that sort of emotional pain is itself a traumatizing experience.

There is a lot of evidence showing finding a support group or therapist can be very helpful in decreasing the chances that you will feel suicidal again in the future. You can get help and referrals from your doctor. Make a wellness recovery action plan (WRAP) by writing down what helps you to feel better about yourself. For example, going for a walk, talking to someone you trust. Or write what helps you get through a crisis and what your distraction techniques includes, such as, a bath with candles, reading and knitting or going for a walk; going for coffee. And learn 'distress tolerance' skills. You should do this when you are well. These skills can help you survive when you're in crisis and support your ongoing mental health. According to professional counselors, Dialectical behavioral therapy (DBT) gives lots of suggestions for accepting distress, soothing yourself and beginning to think more clearly.

In addition, here are ways suggested to cope with suicidal feelings: Online discussions groups can help you to learn practical ways of managing your crisis from others who have been through a similar experience. Unfortunately, the quality of the information and support offered online will vary. In some cases the websites may be harmful if they are not promoting recovery. If you want online support, you could start, for example, by checking my website.

Here are some practical self-help tips: Remove any means of killing yourself because this is important while you learn how to cope with suicidal feelings. For example, make sure that you have only small quantities of medication in the house; if you are no longer driving carefully, hand over your car keys to a friend.

""She who has hope has everything."
--Anonymous--

KEEP MEDICATION LOCKED UP

Experts believe the possibility of suicide is most serious when a person has a plan for committing suicide that includes: having the means, such as weapons or medicines, available to commit suicide or do harm to another person. Or having set a time and place to commit suicide and thinking there is no other way to solve the problem or end the pain. Take any mention of suicide seriously. If someone you know is threatening suicide, get help right away. Health professional should try to find out whether the person has the means (weapons or medicines) available to do harm to themselves or to another person. Or has set a time and place to attempt suicide. Or think that there is no other way to end the pain.

Remember, if a suicide threat seems real, with a specific plan and the means at hand; call 911, a suicide hotline, or the police. Stay with the person, or ask someone you trust to stay with the person, until the crisis has passed. Encourage the person to seek professional help. It's been suggested you don't argue with the person (it's not as bad as you think") or challenge the person (You're not the type to attempt suicide"). Tell the person that you don't want him or her to die, talk about the situation as openly as possible.

There is a lot of evidence showing you can take steps to prevent a suicide attempt. Such as, be willing to listen, and help the person find help; don't be afraid to ask "What is the matter? Or bring up the subject of suicide. There is no evidence that talking about suicide leads to suicidal thinking or suicide. Remove all guns from the home, or lock guns and bullets up in different places. Get rid of any prescription and non-prescription medicines that are not being use.

In addition, it is hard to know if a person is thinking about suicide. Health professionals suggested when watching for warning signs of suicide. You should look for warning signs and events that may make suicide more likely. Study has shown people may be more likely to attempt suicide if they are male; have attempted suicide before, or have had a family member who has killed themselves or who attempted suicide.

Also, have had or have mental health problems such as severe depression, bipolar disorder, schizophrenia, or anxiety. It's also suggested if they have been through family violence, including physical or sexual abuse; drink a lot of alcohol or use drugs. It can also be a veteran or members of the armed services. Here are examples of events that may put people at greater risk for suicide which includes; changes in life such as the death of a partner or good friend, retirement, divorce, or problems with money; the diagnosis of a serious physical illness, such as cancer or heart disease, or a new physical disability, and living alone or not having friends or social contacts.

"The lows were absolutely horrible. It was like falling into a manhole and not being able to lift the lid and climb out."
--Linda Hamilton--

POSITIVE SELF TALK/JOURNAL

Experts believe to help you cope with suicidal thoughts first you must make a list of things you love. This is a list of everything that has helped you cope in the past. Write down the names of your best friends and family members you love, your favorite places, music, movies, books that have save you. Include little things like your favorite foods and sports, bigger things like hobbies and passions that help you wake up in the morning. Also, write down what you love about yourself, your personality traits, physical traits, accomplishments, and things that make you proud. Write down things you plan to do later in life, the places you want to travel, the children you want to have, and people you want to love, experiences you've always wanted. Here are two things to remember when having suicidal thoughts:

1. **Think of all the people who love and care about you.** Though you should not feel guilty for having suicidal thoughts, you can help prevent these thoughts by reminding yourself of all the people in the world who genuinely care about you. Sure, you may be feeling completely alone, but that may be because you've been out of touch with your friends recently or you haven't been feeling close to your family. That doesn't mean that there aren't people who care for you and want you to move forward.

Experts believe, one of the reasons people have suicidal thoughts is because they may feel like no one at all cares about them. Sure, maybe you don't feel like you have any real friendships and you don't have a strong family bond, but that doesn't mean that there's no one who cares for you, even if it's a neighbor, a classmate, or a co-worker. If you're thinking negatively, it's natural to think that absolutely no one cares, but this is rarely the case.

2. **Think of all the things you have yet to do.** This may sound corny, but taking the time to write down and consider all of the things that you haven't done yet, whether it's fall in love or travel to a foreign country, this can give you hope and more of a reason to live. The next time you feel like ending your life, you can think about all of the things you have ahead of you, and you'll see that you have so many more experiences to soak up before your life is over. So smile!

"Your present circumstances don't determine where you can go, they merely determine where you start."
--Nido Qubein--

AVOID DRUGS AND ALCOHOL

If you are using drugs and alcohol while having suicidal thoughts then you should stop. You might be trying to make the thoughts go away by drinking or using drugs. But adding these chemicals to your body actually just makes it a lot harder to think clearly, which you need to be able to do to cope with suicidal thoughts. It's been said drugs and alcohol can make depressive thoughts get out of control. If you're drinking or doing any drugs right now, try to stop to give your mind a break. If you don't feel like you can stop, try being with someone else who don't use drugs or alcohol, just don't stay by yourself.

Health professionals discovered if you're even worrying about preventing suicidal thoughts, then you should avoid drugs and alcohol at all costs. While they may offer a temporary release from your problems, once the effects were off, you will be feeling more depressed and upset than you were to begin with. Both drugs and alcohol are to be avoided at all costs while you're battling with suicidal thoughts; they can also cause you to act impulsively, which is something you definitely want to avoid. Suicidal thoughts can become even stronger if you have taken drugs or alcohol. It is important to not use nonprescription drugs or alcohol when you feel hopeless or are thinking about suicide.

In addition, experts believe suicide is an escalating public health problem, and alcohol use has consistently been implicated in the precipitation of suicidal behavior. It's been said alcohol abuse may lead to sociality through disinhibition, impulsiveness and impaired judgment, but it may also be used as a means to ease the distress associated with committing an act of suicide. The counseling professional reviewed evidence of the relationship between alcohol use and suicide through a search of MedLine and PsychInfo electronic data bases.

It was found, multiple genetically-related intermediate phenotypes might influence the relationship between alcohol and suicide. In addition, Psychiatric disorders, including psychosis, mood disorders and anxiety disorders, as well as susceptibility to stress, might increase the risk of suicidal behavior, but may also have reciprocal influences with alcohol drinking patterns. Increased suicide risk may be signal by social withdrawal, breakdown of social bonds, and social marginalization, which are common outcome of untreated alcohol abuse and dependence. The health professionals feel people with alcohol dependence or depression should be screen for other psychiatric symptoms and for sociality.

And, your programs for suicide prevention must take into account drinking habits and should reinforce healthy behavioral patterns.

"Mental illness is an equal-opportunity illness. Every one of us is impacted by mental illness. One in five adults are dealing with this illness, and many are not seeking help because the stigma prevents that."

--Margaret Larson--

BE MINDFUL

According to Stacey Freedenthal, PhD. LCSW, no matter what you have planned, and what state of mind you're in, you should promise yourself that you'll wait 48 hours or give yourself two days to think things over before you take any action. After everything you've been through, it's really not that much more time to wait. Delaying your plan by 2 day will give you time to sleep on it, talk to people, and figure out if there's any other way to relieve yourself of the pain. Try to separate your thoughts from your actions. You're having suicidal thoughts, but that doesn't mean you have to act on them. It's ok to think one thing and do another. Sometime extreme pain can distort our perception. Waiting before taking action will give your mind time to clear your head.

Too often, people who think of suicide regard their thoughts as truth. They believe them. In a twist on the famous saying "I think, therefore I am," suicide's lie is, "I think I should kill myself, therefore I should kill myself." But it doesn't have to be that way. You can learn to observe your suicidal thoughts without believing them or acting on them by practicing mindfulness says Freedenthal.

The Practice of Mindfulness

Experts define mindfulness in general as a practice that involves observing your thoughts without buying into them. You label your thoughts as just that – thoughts; not necessarily truth and not necessarily a call to action. It's been said if you have the thought, "I should kill myself," you can then observe, "I just had the thought that I should kill myself."

And, if you believe the thought, you might tell yourself, "I believe the thought that I should kill myself." These subtle changes in wording shift the focus from "I should kill myself," a supposed truth to "I think…" or "I am believing…" which in turn highlights that your thought or belief may not be true.

> *"Try it with something innocuous. If you say, "I think I left my keys at home" or "I believe I left my keys at home," that implies doubt. It may or may not be true that you left your keys at home. On the other hand, the statement "I left my keys at home" leaves no doubt that, in fact, your keys are at home."*
> *--Mason Cooley—*

REMAIN CURIOUS

Being curious about your suicidal thoughts is another part of "mindfulness" observation. If you have the thought, "I should kill myself," how does it affect the thought's meaning to then tell yourself, "Hmm, I wonder why I just had the thought that I should kill myself?" Curiosity treats suicidal thoughts for what they are a symptom, not a truth. They are a symptom or a sign that something inside you needs healing. What might that be? Suicidal thoughts can be a symptom of many things. To name just a few, experts believe the cause of suicidal thoughts might be deep emotional pain, an out-of-control addiction, external circumstances that need to change, or a neurochemical imbalance that could respond to medication. In this way, you might respond to suicidal thoughts with the following: "isn't it interesting that I am having the thought that I want to die?' "I wonder why I am having the thought that I want to die." "These thoughts are a symptom. What are they telling me?"

As was previously stated, mindfulness enables you to recognize just how transitory thoughts are. They come and they go, like clouds before the sun. Clouds leave, but the sun is still there. It is always there, even when it is completely hidden by the clouds. The facts show that is how you are. Your true essence is always there, untouched by the suicidal thoughts that may hide it for now. Too often, people who think of suicide regard their thoughts as truth. They believe them.

"I can't change the direction of the wind but I can adjust my sails to always reach my destination."

--Jimmy Dean--

BE SAFE

If you are having suicidal thoughts the first thing you should do is make your home safer. Since you've made a promise to yourself to wait, keep yourself safe in the meantime. Put away anything that you could use to harm yourself, like pills, razors, sharp objects, guns and give them to someone else for safekeeping or toss them out or lock them away. Don't make it easy for yourself to change your mind. If you don't feel safe staying by yourself at home, go to a place where you do feel safe, like a friend's house, your parent's house, or a community center or other public place. Professional counselors have said suicidal intentions are prompted by a desperate need for relief from intensely painful feelings. Study has shown, surviving having suicidal thoughts is about learning how to find relief without resorting to suicide. Simply having suicidal thoughts does not mean you will act on them. However, the habit of repeatedly thinking about suicide is a risky one because repetition brings a sense of falsely comforting familiarity. Health professions believe it dulls the instinctive recoil from danger. Although it may be difficult, hold on to the belief that there ARE ways to resist depression and find relief.

In addition, health professionals suggest you prepare a safety plan. It helps you plan ahead for the times when you may feel particularly low and at risk of acting on your suicidal thoughts. It is a way to personalize and summaries the possible strategies for taking care of you.

Also, a Safety Plan supports your healthier self (the part of you that wants to hold on and survive) when things are hard and you are feeling overwhelmed.

The health professionals list 3 strategies that will offer a solid foundation for creating a safety plan and for working toward breaking the suicidal thinking habit:

1. **Make a commitment to yourself:** When you notice thoughts of suicide, challenge the self-bulling habit and make a commitment to taking care of yourself as best you possibly can for the moment. Remind yourself to follow your safety plan if you have made one, or you can use the general safety plan set out of the "Feeling like you want to die?"

2. **Attend to yourself care needs:** Suicidal thoughts arise as a result of deeply painful feelings of despair and hopelessness. Recognize the pain you are feeling as something which needs a compassionate and caring response. Practice constructive ways to take care of yourself when you are feeling this way.

3. **Tell someone how you're feeling:** Tell someone else how you are feeling or get someone to be with you. Be prepared for nonprofessionals to be shocked by what you tell them, and don't expect a perfect response; it is always better to make human contact than you stay isolated and alone with your thoughts.

"Not until we are lost do we begin to understand ourselves."
--Henry David Thoreau--

HOW TO REDUCE THE RISKS

When you are having suicidal thoughts protect yourself from impulsively acting on your thoughts by putting dangerous objects out of immediate reach. Preferably give pills, weapons etc to someone else for safe-keeping, but even putting them in a locked or inaccessible place makes it a little harder to act impulsively.

Also, plan to get professional help. It is unreasonable to see suicide as the only solution if you haven't sought any professional help for your depression and suicidal thinking. Doctors and counselors help many people move on from depression so get the appropriate help you need. And, you may need to challenge yourself about what's stopping you from getting help.

Next, check medication side effects. There is a lot of evidence showing some anti-depressant medication can increase the risk of suicidal thinking, especially when you first start taking them so be aware. Also, doctors say when the medication first starts taking effect it can increase your energy and motivation before improving your mood, increasing the risk of acting on suicidal thoughts so talk to your doctor about the risks and be open with other strategies for keeping yourself safe.

In addition, check alcohol and drugs. As mention before, both alcohol and drugs tend to reduce your inhibitions and make it more likely you could do something you will regret the next day. Check your alcohol/drug consumption and try to cut down. Also, try not to drink alone or to end up alone after drinking you need to minimize time spent alone because depression and suicidal thinking thrive in isolation. Try to minimize time spent alone in your room by taking work to the library, ask friends to be with you at vulnerable times, make plans ahead for weekends and other lonelier times, and work on building your support networks. Also, though you feel like withdrawing, ask trusted friends and acquaintances to spend time with you. Or continue to call a crisis helpline and talk about your feelings. Develop a set of steps that you can follow during a suicidal crisis. It should include contact numbers for your doctor or therapist, as well as friends and family members who will help in an emergency. Make a written schedule for yourself every day and stick to it, no matter what. Keep a regular routine as much as possible, even when your feelings seem out of control. Get out in the sun or into nature for at least 30 minutes a day. Exercise as vigorously as is safe for you to get the most benefit, aim for 30 minutes of exercise per day. But you can start small. Three 10-minute bursts of activity can have a positive effect on mood. Make time for things that bring you joy even if very few things bring you pleasure at that moment; force yourself to do the things you used to enjoy.

And, remember your personal goals. You may have always wanted to travel to particular place, read a specific book, own a pet, move to another place, learn a new hobby, volunteer, go back to school, or start a family. Write your personal goals down.

"You, yourself, as much as anybody in the entire universe, deserve your love and affection."

--The Buddha--

GIVE YOURSELF SMALL GOALS

Before or while you are having suicidal thoughts each evening set yourself a small tasks or goals for the next day. It can be something as simple as watching a certain TV programmed. Or set yourself another task as soon as you have completed one. Just knowing you can still do things you set for yourself despite feeling low can help combat depression and allow you to identify depressed thinking habits.

It's been said suicidal thinking is the ultimate all-or-nothing thinking habit, and the culmination of other habits of depressed thinking which intensify the depression habit spiral. Learn more about identifying and challenging depressed thinking, particularly self bullying and start breaking the suicidal thinking habit. We can't stop thoughts from entering our heads, but we can stop actively inviting them in. Try to stop using thoughts of suicide as a barometer for how bad you are feeling. Use self soothing or distraction techniques (such as what was mentioned) when you notice thoughts about suicide bothering you, practice other techniques (that are found in this book) for challenging depressed thinking.

In addition, understand some of the reasons for suicidal thinking because suicide is such a taboo, you may not be aware of how common it is for people to think about suicide and of the various general reasons for suicidal thinking. Read 'Thinking about suicide' and 'Making sense of suicide' and assess your own suicidal thinking habit to identify which reasons are relevant to you.

Also, work on rebuilding meaning in your life because depression works to drain assumed meaning out of life and challenges us to take responsibility for making our lives meaningful.

Challenge the distrust or perfectionism which may be preventing you from embracing hopeful or constructive ideals and goals for your life

"I think you have to try and fail, because failure gets you closer to what you're good at."

--Louis C.K.--

Chapter 13

COMMUNICATION

Communication is one of the most frequent activities we do on a day-to-day basis. You may have felt, as we all have at some time or other, that you were not communicating as well as you would have liked especially if you have a mental health diagnosis. The goal of this chapter is to help you assess your skills for discussing your thoughts, feelings, needs and problems. You may find that you are already using the kinds of communication we are going to discuss. If so, you are on the right track. The communication tips are useful for everyone in your family, including your family member living with mental illness. Good communication may improve relationships between your family member and health professionals as well.

In addition, mental illness can create additional communication challenges. Even at the best of times it can be difficult to talk about sensitive topics. Sometimes communicating with your family members will be one of the hardest things you do. Good communication can help to; express concerns and worries you may have about your family member in a non-threatening way. Communication can also reduce the risk of relapse by creating a positive environment at home. So try to improve communication with health professionals involved in your family member's care and clarify what each member of your family can do to help in your family member's recovery journey.

To add, while I have thoroughly enjoyed writing about my experience in mental health techniques, your ultimate aim may be to share your story in front of a group of people as I do.

I know words and writing can be extremely powerful, but I truly believe that writing does "lose" some of its emotional power if you can't see the expressions on the persons face. And, we know that we can often misinterpret things written on face book, via text or email because you might take "words the wrong way", so you really want to be able to speak openly to people about your experiences to add depth, power, and personality so that people know they have talk to a real person, who has truly lived this experience and survived, and not some computer generated person who is someone making up their story. Some people will hid behind their ipad and text messages while writing, and can shelter their tears and emotions from other people view, but it's time to step out of your comfort zone and begin to talk, face to face, about your experience.

Lastly, we will look at each type of communication in more detail in this chapter. Let's start with communicating face to face. In face to face we have all the cues available to us: words, facial expression, gestures, body language, tone of voice, room temperature, room noise, and other people in the room that might be present. If there is something missing in the person's words, or if a person is trying to hide how they feel there are other cues that will complement the message, if they are congruent with the words. The message will be more complete and clear when all cues are present and most of the times they are if you look close enough.

LONG DISTANCE COMMUNICATIONS

Experts believe videoconferencing and web conferencing are almost as effective as face to face communication. The only cue that is missing in video and web conferencing is the shared presence or surroundings that may give people additional information about the message meaning. And telephone communication lacks nonverbal cues. When we are having a phone conversation, we don't have facial expressions or body language to help us decode messages, so we must focus on every word being said, and the tone of voice that is being used. It's been said we compensate for the absence of nonverbal cues by adding more weight to the words being said and the tone of voice being used. The remaining types of communication on the chart are missing both, tone of voice as well as nonverbal communication. They only use words and visuals. Does that mean that the quality of the communication is minimal? Not necessarily, it means that the words and visuals carry all the weight to ensure a message is clearly understood.

It is said texting or instant messaging communication can be a place where people hide who do not know how to express themselves. When we text each other using a phone or a cell phone, we only have words to send our message and to receive it. We are missing tone of voice, facial expressions, body language and presence to help us decode the message (a person could say or be anywhere). To complicate matters, when we text we use shorthand (e.g. LOL for laughing out loud). We also misspell or shorten words because we don't want to use a tiny space to write long messages, and because we're in a rush to send the messages out. After all, it's instant messaging, not for holding a long conversation on (like most people try to do who are afraid to speak face-to-face or use the phone to talk with people).

In addition, communicating experts said, email is equivalent to texting, (it's know better when it comes to communicating) with an added disadvantage: In email communication there is a delay in between messages being sent, received and replied to and this prevents a solid thread in the conversation from forming. When someone sends you an email, they are in a frame of mind that may or may not be the same later, or when you read and reply to their email. Your reply is now floating in a different time, it may link to the original message or it may be irrelevant who knows. The same applies to your reply, there may be a delay between the time you send it and the time the other person reads it.

Also, communication experts feel postal mail is very similar to email communication, with an added disadvantage as well. The message takes longer to reach its intended recipient and is less convenient to write and send. Now you have paper, pens, envelopes and stamps to find. You may write less often. Traditional mail has a subjective value over email. It is said people think of traditional mail as more personal when compared to email. Seeing the person's scribbling on the page is appealing and personal because you recognize the writing; you know the sender took the time to write you, so you may hang on to every word with more attention than ever.

"It is during our darkest moments that we most focus to see the light."

--Aristotle Onassis--

LETTER

Let's show how writing a letter instead of email can help with your recovery. For some people, it may take some time for them to adjust and continue to recover after experiencing a psychiatric crisis, especially if they were hospitalized. Recovery is an ongoing process that takes time and patience.

For example, while you recover after a crisis, you may need to communicate to your friends and family that you need a lot of rest. At this time, you may not be able to deal with their demands and expectations of you. They may think that now that the crisis is over, everything should be back to normal and it may be hard to convince them that you need rest to get your strength back and that this phase may last awhile. Below is two example of a letter that is suggested by communication experts to use to let your friends and family know what you need during this time. This is just guidance and you can certainly rewrite it to fit your circumstances and style. Dear Friends and Family, "I am writing this letter to ask for your understanding, compassion and patience. We have all just come through a difficult time with my mental health condition. I realize that this has not been easy for you and you have likely struggled to deal with its effects while continuing to take care of yourself and others. It has not been easy for any of us. I have done the best I could and I know you have too." For this, I thank you.

In addition, a similar example could state, as a result of this experience, I am exhausted, physically and mentally. I may look all right on the outside, but inside I am still hurting. I need time to recuperate and recover. Please understand that even the least effort or stress is difficult for me right now. I need to sleep a lot, and not do much at all. I need this time to regain my strength and I am not sure how long it will last. It may be hard for you to see me this way.

You may feel it is your duty to help me get over this. Please know that neither of these is true. Please be gentle and work with me because I need time to heal. I understand this has been difficult for you too, but I believe if we work together as a team, we can all heal and recover from this traumatic experience. Here are a few things you can do to help me: Learn about my mental health condition, help me find effective treatment, and listen with an open heart and mind. Thank you for your support; it makes all the difference in my journey of recovery.

    These examples can be uses for any type of recovery by exchanging the words to express how you feel.

"Out of suffering have emerged the strongest souls; the most massive characters are seared with scars."

--Khalil gibrun--

BODY LANGUAGE

Body language affects how others see us, but it may also change how we see ourselves. Social psychologist Amy Cuddy shows how "power posing" standing in a posture of confidence, even when we don't feel confident, can affect testosterone and cortical levels in the brain, and might even have an impact on our chances for success. Body language and non-verbal communications are vague. The Oxford English Dictionary defines body language as the conscious and unconscious movements and postures by which attitudes and feelings are communicated.

For example, "her intent was clearly expressed in her body language." Body language certainly also include where the body is in relation to other bodies (often referred to as personal space). Body language also includes very small bodily movements such as facial expressions and eye movements. Social experts also believe body language arguably covers all that we communicate through our bodies apart from the spoken words (thereby encompassing breathing, perspiration, pulse, blood-pressure, blushing, etc.). "Body language is the unconscious and conscious transmission and interpretation of feelings, attitudes, and moods, through: body posture, movement, physical state, position and relationship to other bodies, objects and surroundings, facial expression and eye movement."

In addition, when we interact with others, we continuously give and receive wordless signals. All of our nonverbal behaviors and the gestures we make, such as, the way we sit, how fast or how loud we talk, how close we stand, how much eye contact we make all send strong messages. These messages don't stop when you stop speaking either. Even when you're silent, you're still communicating nonverbally. Oftentimes, what comes out of our mouths and what we communicate through our body language are two totally different things. When faced with these mixed signals, the listener has to choose whether to believe your verbal or nonverbal message, and, in most cases, they're going to choose the nonverbal because it's a natural, unconscious language that broadcasts our true feelings and intentions in any given moment. Also, the way you listen, look, move, and react tells the other person whether or not you care, if you're being truthful, and how well you're listening. When your nonverbal signals match up with the words you're saying, they increase trust, clarity, and rapport. On the other hand, when they don't, they generate tension, mistrust, and confusion (most people don't know their body is at work as well as their mouth.) If you want to become a better communicator, it's important to become more sensitive not only to the body language and nonverbal cues of others, but also to yourself. Stay true to yourself and others and you can't go wrong.

"You alone are enough. You have nothing to prove to anybody."

--Maya Angelou--

NONVERBAL COMMUNICATION ROLES

Communication experts believe the role of nonverbal communication is to repeat the message the person is making verbally; it can contradict a message the individual is trying to convey; or it can substitute for a verbal message. For example, a person's eyes can often convey a far more vivid message than words do. Nonverbal communication can also add to or complement a verbal message. For example, a boss who pats a person on the back in addition to giving praise can increase the impact of the message. It can accent or underline a verbal message. Or pounding the table, for example, can underline a message. For more information on nonverbal read, "The Importance of Effective Communication," by Edward G. Wertheim, Ph.D.

According to Wertheim there are many different types of nonverbal communication, together, the following nonverbal signals and cues communicate your interest and investment in others. Such as facial expressions, the human face is extremely expressive, able to express countless emotions without saying a word. And unlike some forms of nonverbal communication, facial expressions are universal. The facial expressions for happiness, sadness, anger, surprise, fear, and disgust are the same across cultures.

In addition, consider how your perceptions of people are affected by the way they sit, walk, stand up, or hold their head. The way you move and carry youself can communicate a wealth of information to the world. This type of nonverbal communication includes your posture, bearing, stance, and subtle movements. Also, it is said, gestures are woven into the fabric of our daily lives. We wave, point, beckon, and use our hands when we're arguing or speaking animatedly, expressing ourselves with gestures often without thinking.

However, the meaning of gestures can be very different across cultures and regions, so it's important to be careful to avoid misinterpretation.

Lastly, since the visual sense is dominant for most people, eye contact is an especially important type of nonverbal communication. The way you look at someone can communicate many things, including interest, affection, hostility, or attraction. Eye contact is also important in maintaining the flow of conversation and for engaging the other person's response.

"To be ill adjusted to a deranged world is not a breakdown."
--Jeanette Winterson--

COMMUNICATION THROUGH TOUCH

We communicate a great deal through touch. Think about the messages given by something as little as a weak handshake, a timid tap on the shoulder, a warm bear hug, a reassuring slap on the back, a patronizing pat on the head, or a controlling grip on your arm. I am sure we all have experience one of the above touch.

And, have you ever felt uncomfortable during a conversation because the other person was standing too close and invading your space? We all have a need for physical space, although that need differs depending on the culture, the situation, and the closeness of the relationship. You can use physical space to communicate many different nonverbal messages, including signals of intimacy and affection, aggression or dominance says self-esteem counseling professionals.

In addition, it's not just what you say it's how you say it. When we speak, other people "read" our voices as well as listen to our words. Here are a few things communication experts suggest people to do. Pay attention to it include your timing and pace, how loud you are speaking, your tone and inflection, and the sounds that convey understanding, such as "ahh" and "uh-huh." Think about how someone's tone of voice can indicate sarcasm, anger, affection, or confidence. I always depend on my nonverbal communication skill when talking to someone because I know nonverbal communication can't be faked. You may be familiar with advice you received on how to sit a certain way, steeple your fingers or shake hands just to appear confident or assert dominance. But the truth is that such tricks aren't likely to work (unless you truly feel confident and in charge). That's because you can't control all of the signals you're constantly sending off about what you're really thinking and feeling says counseling professionals. And the harder you try, the more unnatural your signals are likely to come across to others. Remember, touch is not a widely used form of communication in western society; we are not a "touchy-feely" society. Touch is usually reserved for our most intimate relationships and for communication between close friends. Although it is acceptable for women to touch in public, many believe it is not 'proper' for men to do so. Sadly, even in the privacy of your home, a son may be embarrassed when he is embraced by his father,

    And, many are a little surprised when we see pictures of men in other countries embracing or walking arm in arm. It is important for you to remember when communicating with people from other countries and other cultures that their nonverbal communications differ from yours just as their language may be unlike yours. Touching may be a very acceptable and a very common form of nonverbal communication in the country where you are transacting business; you should understand this and be prepared for it.

> *"Here is the test to find whether your mission on earth is finished; if you're alive it isn't."*
>
> *--Richard Bach--*

HUMOR FOR COMMUNICATION AND PERSUASION

Humor has many benefits for communication and persuasion. Here are just a few. Studies by Fabio Sala at the Hay Group have shown that humor (used skillfully) reduces hostility, deflects criticism, relieves tension, improves morale, helps communicate difficult messages. Other research by Bettinghaus and Cody (1994) and Food (1997) showed that humor, builds rapport and liking of the humorist, makes the target person want to listen more, relaxes the person, making them more receptive to the message, makes the person feel good and there for not think so carefully about the proposition. It also makes the information more memorable, and distracts the person from thinking about counter-arguments. This is especially important in situations where the initial mood of the conversation is hostile or confrontational.

Also, research has shown humor in this situation helps reduce hostile feelings among co-workers and partners. When you're in a better mood that shared laughter provides it puts you in a better position to resolve the conflict and get on with your job. It is a fact that humor and laughter are incompatible with anger and other negative emotions that's why it makes humor such a great tool for conflict management. Since conflict and stress are so common in the workplace these days, the savvy manager will cultivate appropriately-timed humor as a means of keeping tensions, frustration and upset from escalating to lay the foundation for better communication.

In addition, humor plays an important role when persuading someone to do something you want them to do. There is several persuasion theories used to persuade someone. Humor can be incorporated into these persuasion theories and may or may not help you persuade someone.

Humor may help you persuade someone or back fire on you. The most important thing to remember when using humor is to know when to use it in your argument and when not to use it. It is said, if you are successful in using humor to persuade someone you will be able to establish good rapport with them and you will be like and respected. People will want to hear more of what you have to say and will be more easily persuaded by you.

On the other hand, if you use humor at an inappropriate time in your argument you could risk the possibility of offending the person you are trying to persuade. Knowing when and when not to use humor in persuasion will ensure you have greater success when it comes to persuading someone into doing something you want them to do.

"Never let the opinions of others become the measure of your self-worth."

--Healthline--

LISTEN

According to research the importance of listening in communication is enormous. People often focus on their speaking ability believing that good speaking equals good communication. The ability to speak well is a necessary component to successful communication and the ability to listen is equality as important. The importance of listening in communication is often well illustrated when we analyze our listen skills with those closest to us. In particular I am referring to our spouse, partner, children or friends. Pay attention to the everyday conversations we have with these people with whom we think we communicate well. Communication is essential for all individuals to make their needs, wants and ideas known and with a mental health diagnosis, communication skills may be delayed or wrought with difficulties. Developing skills to work with the communication deficits and delays in an individual will improve the quality of their lives.

In addition, listening is one of the most important aspects of effective communication. Communication experts believe successful listening means not just understanding the words or the information being communicated, but also understanding how the speaker feels about what they're communicating. Effective listening can make the speaker feel heard and understood which can help build a stronger, deeper connection between you and the speaker. So create an environment where everyone feels safe to express ideas, opinions, and feelings, or plan and problem solve in creative ways.

Also, you can save time by helping clarify information, avoid conflicts and misunderstandings. When emotions are running high, if the speaker feels that he or she has been truly heard, it can help to calm them down, relieve negative feelings, and allow for real understanding or problem solving to begin.

This will relieve negative emotions and relax the person who is speaking.

"The thing about people who truly and malignantly crazy: their real genius is for making the people around them think they themselves are crazy. In military science this is called Psy-Ops, for your info."

--David Foster Wallace--

KEEP VOICE EVEN

There is a lot of evidence showing communication involves so much more than merely speaking. No matter what you say, your voice makes the difference in how others perceive and interpret your words. This is way using a strong voice when communicating is important. The tone you use, your pitch, and even something as simple as an appropriate pause can communicate more to your listeners than all of the carefully crafted dialogue in the world. So speak up, do not raise your voice to the point of irritation, but simply speak loudly, clearly and confidently to make a good impression. A soft-spoken voice can often suggest timid or uncertainty, so project your voice when you speak. Experts believe when you lower you pitch slightly it command respect. While this holds true for men slightly more than women, even a woman can generate more attention and respect by speaking in a slightly lower pitch. Also, adjust the speed of your voice according to your message. It's been said you can energize people by speaking more quickly, and build suspense by speaking more slowly. In essence, the speed at which you speak has the power to impact the mood of the conversation and ultimately guide the emotional responses of those listening. You can take a brief pause from time to time. If you say something that needs time to sink in, or if you want to allow time for response, do not hesitate to pause. Watch you inflections. Emphasize the words most pertinent to your message and vary your inflections from sentence to sentence. This lets people know that you have something interesting and meaningful to say, as opposed to the monotone speaker who bores listeners to death with his robotic speech.

In addition, the facts show words are often very imprecise vehicles of communication, requiring us to be as highly reliant on how a person sounds and expresses when communicating. Of course, your voice and themselves expressions is a very powerful tool for communicating when used properly, and a friendly tone of voice can make you seem more approachable and kind, and it might even make some new friends. What makes a voice sound friendly? A "friendly" voice lets people know that they can trust, rely upon, and be reassured by you. This will usually involve speaking clearly, naturally, with confidence, and without any nerves constricting your voice. On the other hand, the opposite of a friendly voice would include shouting or yelling, speaking too quickly, mumbling, and sounding urgent or irritated. The best way to sound friendly is to speak from the heart.

"Mental health is sickness just like diabetes, heart problems, eye problems, we all need help."

--Bettie Jordon--

PROPER LANGUAGE

Using proper language is a skill worth developing to help us to communicate using well-structured language that will enhance clarity of expression. A word loosely spoken can lose a friend or even cause a war. Even in modern times there are some among us who do not care much about what they say or write. They react when an impulse moves. Then they alter words that come to their mind without thinking of the effect that such loosely spoken work would have on others. Unusually, a bad word is sharp like the sharp ended knife or a sword.

Also, there are other words that can resemble blades with extreme sharpness at both edges. For this reason it is true to say that, the tongue is like a sharp knife and it can kill without drawing blood. "The ability to communicate is not the same thing as the ability to use "proper" grammar; knowing proper grammar merely allows you to express ideas in ways that are acceptable to a certain class of people, or to control the meaning of grammar to convey things faintly." But communication skills can be quite good even if one's grammar isn't perfect (or if one isn't a native speaker of the language in question). Communicative competence means someone has the ability to make him or she understood, despite technical shortcomings in grammar. Remember, good grammar is not a prerequisite for communicative competence.

In addition, communication experts believe grammar is an important essence to communication because it helps structure our sentences and it can help in how well we communicate. One who has good writing (grammar: "syntax", "pragmatic", "semantics") is an effective communicator because they will usually be able to catch on to the social rules which help us communicate. On the other hand, if one has poor grammar, they will not be able to communicate effectively, (they will say the wrong things or not make sense to the speaker), some grammar errors are okay during communication but some aren't, such as saying "Hey how's it going", that sounds right but when you say "going hey how's it" notice how they do not make any sense, the other speaker may reply with (depending on how you communicate). And, notice how using improper grammar can have an impact on social communication skills, it makes it harder to socially communicate with someone that's why when we get in communication situations whether it's with a client or someone you know, that's why you have to use proper grammar because the listener may get annoyed with you and walk away or because of an misunderstanding make fun of you.

> *"The world I believe in is one where we're measured by our ability to overcome adversities. Not avoid them."*
>
> *--Kevin Breel--*

COMMUNICATE WITH LOVE

Research show many of you do not understand or have forgotten how to communicate with love. You spend your time communicating out of anger and fear in every communication you have, whether it be with a loved one, a partner, a child, or a friend. The emotions of fear and anger do not make for truthful or light communication and it puts you in a space of negativity and fear. Many are fearful and are anxious as to how their communication will come across. Many are afraid of being rejected or laughed at and wonder if they should express truthfully their love. Also, many live their lives in this space and never enter into a truthful conversation because they fear the pain.

But study has shown once there is loving communication you will be in a place of love and will only feel love. This may be hard for many of you to understand because you have always been taught and shown to hide your emotions and to hold back on expressing love. You are loving beings and you go against yourself and the Divine by not expressing yourself in loving ways and especially through communicating. You hold back on expressing your love and expressing yourself because of fear, again, the higher vibrations no longer tolerate fear based emotions. It is time to let go of that "old" way of being and to embrace the loving spirit that you truly are. Everyone's relationship is unique, and people come together for many different reasons. But there are some things that good relationships have in common and that is are love. It's been said knowing the basic principles of healthy relationships helps keep them meaningful, fulfilling and exciting in both happy times and sad.

In addition, some relationships get stuck in peaceful coexistence, but without truly relating to each other and working together. While it may seem stable on the surface, lack of involvement and communication increases distance and when you do need to talk about something important, the connection and understanding may no longer be there. Some couples talk things out quietly, while others may raise their voices and passionately disagree.

     According to relationship experts, when it comes to relationships do not be fearful of conflict. You need to be safe to express things that bother you without fear of retaliation, and be able to resolve conflict without humiliation, degradation or insisting on being right. And remember no one person can meet all of our needs, and expecting too much from someone can put a lot of unhealthy pressure on a relationship. Having friends and outside interests not only strengthens your social network, but brings new insights and stimulation to the relationship as well. Honest, direct communication is a key part of any relationship. When both people feel comfortable expressing their needs, fears, and desires, trust and bonds are strengthened. It's been said nonverbal cues, body language like eye contact, leaning forward or away, or touching someone's arm, are critical to communication.

"Everything has beauty but not everyone sees it."
--Confucius--

KEEP PHYSICAL INTIMACY ALIVE

Relationship experts suggest touching is a fundamental part of human existence. Studies on infants have shown the importance of regular, loving touch and holding on brain development. These benefits do not end in childhood. Life without physical contact with others is a lonely life indeed. Studies have shown that affectionate touch actually boosts the body's levels of oxytocin, a hormone that influences bonding and attachment. In a committed relationship between two adult partners, physical intercourse is often a cornerstone of the relationship. However, intercourse should not be the only method of physical intimacy in a relationship. Regular, affectionate such as holding hands, hugging, or kissing is equally important. While touch is a key part of a healthy relationship, it's important to take some time to find out what your partner really likes. Unwanted touching or inappropriate overtures can make the other person tense up and retreat and that is exactly what you don't want.

Relationship experts, advice these 2 tips: One, spend quality time together. You probably have fond memories of when you were first dating your loved one. Everything may have seemed new and exciting, and you may have spent hours just chatting together or coming up with new, exciting things to try. However, as time goes by, children, demanding jobs, long commutes, different hobbies and other obligations can make it hard to find time together. It's critical for your relationship, though, to make time for yourselves because if you don't have quality time, communication with others can be unsuccessful.

Two, express your feelings. Try to be, specific rather than general about how you feel. Consistently using only one or two words to say how you are feeling, such as bad or upset is too vague and general. State what kind of bad or upset you are such as irritated, mad, anxious, afraid, sad, hurt, lonely, etc. Specify the degree of the feelings, and you will reduce the chances of being misunderstood. For example, some people may think when you say, "I am angry" means you are extremely angry when you actually mean a "little irritated". When expressing anger or irritation, first describe the specific behavior you don't like, then your feelings. This helps to prevent the other person from becoming immediately defensive or intimidated when he first hears "I am angry with you", and he/she could miss the message. If you have mixed feelings, say so, and express each feeling and explain what each feeling is about. For example: "I have mixed feelings about what you just did. I am glad and thankful that you helped me, but I didn't like the comment about being stupid. It was disrespectful and unnecessary and I found it irritating".

"Everyday is a new beginning, treat it that way. Stay away from what might have been and move on. Don't let negative words or actions of others affect your smile. Decide that today is going to be good day."

--rawforbeauty--

EXPRESSING FEELINGS

Communication experts suggest the two following "I feel statements" and "I messages" will help you express feelings productively. Respectfully confront someone when you are bothered by his or her behavior by expressing difficult feelings without attacking the self-esteem of the person; clarify for your understanding and the other person precisely what you feel; prevent feelings from building up and festering into a bigger problem.

And, communicate difficult feelings in a manner that minimizes the other person's need to become defensive, and increases the likelihood that the person will listen. When you first start using these techniques (like anything new) they will be cumbersome and awkward to apply, and not very useful if you only know them as techniques.

However, if you practice these techniques and turn them into skills, it will be easy for you to express difficult feelings in a manner that is productive and respectful. The methods use for expressing your feelings should depend on your goal, the importance or difficulty of your feelings and the situation.

In addition, here are some "I" techniques you can use to develop coping skill for a better communication. The "I feel statements" take the form of "when you did that thing, I felt this way, that thing is a behavior of the other person, and this way is your specific feelings. Here is some example of "I" statements, "I felt embarrassed when you told our friends how we are pinching pennies." "I liked it when you helped with the dishes without being asked." "I feel hurt and am disappointed that you forgot our anniversary."

I Messages are called I message because the focus is on you, and the message is message which focused on and gives a message about the other person. When using "I" messages you take responsibility for your own feelings, rather than accusing the other person of making you feel a certain way. And, your message does not communicate a feeling, but a belief about the other person. The essence of your "I" message is "I have a problem", while the essence of a "You" message is "You have a problem." Experts believe there are four parts to an "I message: "When...describe the person's behavior you are reacting to in an objective, non-blameful, and non-judgmental manner. The effects are...describing the concrete or tangible effects of that behavior. (This is the most important part for the other person to understand, your reaction.) I feel... say how you feel. (This is the most important part to prevent a buildup of feelings.) I'd prefer...Tell the person what you want or what you prefer they do. You can omit this part if it is obvious.

"Nothing defines the quality of life in a community more clearly than people who regard themselves, or whom the consensus chooses to regard, as mentally unwell."
--Renata Adler--

AGREE TO DISAGREE

A good way to end this chapter is to discuss how to agree to disagree. Instead of getting heated and arguing until you are blue in the face, keep telling yourself to agree to disagree on certain topics. This way you can have lively debates without letting them get personal. Be a good sport. In an argument or debate, keep a friendly mind-set. Though some issues may be incredibly important to you, like your religious beliefs, understand that everyone has the right to their own opinion. If everyone believed the same thing life would get boring. Stay calm in the face of a debate. Agree to disagree with someone who is able to intelligently converse with you about tough subjects. Keep your cool and simply swap ideas with this person instead of letting it get ugly. Use honestly above all. People will tend to throw up their hands and plead that there is no winning or losing the argument when they have clearly lost. This tends to happen to those who have not fully researched or thoughts out their opinion on the subject.

In addition, respect the other person. In a debate, friendly or otherwise, if the person states that you should just agree to disagree, accept it, even if you think they are saying so to avoid admitting defeat. Understand that you can't change a mind that does not want to change. Some people will be open to new ways to thinking, and others are steadfast in their beliefs and cling to them as though their lives depended on it. Take this fact to heart, and it will help you be a better debater. Even in the strongest of relationships, there will be times when small irritations can cause mountains to grow out of molehills, so it's important to keep striving for better communication.

To add, communication has a great impact on every aspect of life. Yet the channels of communication can sometimes become blocked, even among people who care deeply for each other. It's often difficult to put our feelings into words or concentrate fully when our partner speaks. Unhelpful silences or verbal attacks can arise and drive us further apart. Communication experts feel some of the common barriers people will face will include, threatening or unpleasant behavior such as criticism and bossiness; only hearing what we want to hear; getting bored or distracted; and not expressing our point clearly. Fortunately, working on our communication skills helps us to break through this sort of impasse. So follow these tried and tested tips to stop you reaching for the expletives and reach an understanding instead. No matter what else is going on, try to make time for your partner on a day-to-day basis. Good communication is about deepening your understanding of each other, not simply avoiding arguments. Easier said than done, of course, but making time to talk is worth the effort.

    All being well, these occasions will be enjoyable and bring great rewards, so make a dinner date, share a bath or go for a walk together and let the conversation flow. Secondly, remember the importance of intimate, non-sexual contact. Hugs and kisses are the glue which holds a relationship together, and consider activities such as sport to reconnect non-verbally. Psychologist believes the vast majority of communicating takes place without words through body language.

> "Schizophrenia cannot be understood without understanding despair."
>
> --R. D. Laing--

Chapter 14

FLASHBACKS

According to The National Institute of Mental Health, a flashback, or involuntary recurrent memory, is a psychological phenomenon in which an individual has a sudden, usually powerful, re-experiencing or a past experience or elements of a past experience. These experiences can be happy, sad, exciting, or any other emotion one can consider.

It's been said, the term is used particularly when the memory is recalled involuntarily, and/or when it is so intense that the person "relives" the experience, unable to fully recognize it as memory and not something that is happening in "real time". Also, flashbacks are the "personal experiences that pop into your awareness, without any conscious, premeditated attempt to search and retrieve this memory." These experiences sometimes have little to no relation to the situation at hand. Flashbacks to those suffering posttraumatic stress disorder can be so disruptive as to seriously affect day-to-day living. Experts believe, memory is divided into voluntary (conscious) and involuntary (unconscious) processes that function independently of each other.

In addition, doctors suggest flashbacks are often associated with mental illness as they are a symptom and a feature in diagnostic criteria for posttraumatic stress disorder (PTSD), acute stress disorder, and obsessive-compulsive disorder (OCD). There is evidence showing flashbacks have also been observed in people suffering from manic depression, depression, homesickness, near-death experiences, epileptic seizures, and drug abuse. Some researchers have suggested that the use of some drugs can cause a person to experience flashbacks. Users of lysergic acid diethylamide sometimes report "acid flashbacks". While other studies show that the use of drugs, specifically cannabis, can help reduce the occurrence of flashbacks in people with PTSD.

Also, the psychological phenomenon has frequently been portrayed in film and television. Some of the most accurate media portrayals of flashbacks have been those related to wartime, and the association of flashbacks to Post-traumatic Stress Disorder cause by the traumas and stress of war. One of the earliest screen portrayals of this is in the 1945 film Mildred Pierce.

WRITE DOWN THE MEMORY/EVENTS OF THE INCIDENT

Study has shown it is very important to take notes of the flashback. Whether you simply make mental notes or write down every detail about the flashback and what you did to cope, this is an important part of the process. Experts believe, the more information you have about your flashbacks, the better you become in dealing with it. Try to write down what triggered the flashback; what was your goal (accept, control or escape); did you accomplish your goal; what coping techniques did you use; and which of these techniques helped, which didn't. Having these notes can help create a better plan for flashback management. They can also help your therapist in helping you control your flashbacks.

The facts show, nearly anything you can do to help cope with your flashbacks is a good thing. I say nearly everything because anything that does harm to yourself or another person is simply inexcusable in my opinion. Doctors suggest, when you are alone try to play memory games, it is said one of the easiest ways to cope or manage a flashback is by distraction. Try to remember something challenging such as the lyrics to a particular song, or a favorite poem. This can help interrupt the flashback by redirecting the activity in your brain. For some reason, memory games work well when you have flashbacks that involved hearing and balance. Some of the more effective memory games are humming songs or remembering the lyrics to songs and Naming facts you learned in school.

In addition, there is a lot of evidence that show, using ice cubes has been the most important tool in dealing with physically oriented flashbacks. The idea is simple says the counseling profession; you take a fairly large ice cube and hold it tight in one of your hands throughout the flashback.

The cold feeling keeps the part of you grounded to some degree and the physical sensation gives you something solid to focus on besides the memory you are reliving. It is important to hold the ice cube fairly tight and in the same hand for the duration of the flashback. Another technique is called wall spotting, this technique involves selecting 4 or 5 brightly colored items in the room that are easily within vision and moving your focus between them. Make sure to vary the order, it allows you to lock onto the items briefly before shifting to the next item. Most people with flashbacks reported, you should keep this up throughout the flashback and continue for a short time afterwards. Following the same pattern can actually cause you to become more involved in the flashback because your mind becomes used to the pattern and build on it.

It is said, by varying the pattern, you disrupt the thought processes involved in the flashback. Also, try cold on your face; again this is a simple and can help with any type of flashback. This idea is use and reported to be one of the first ones you find that helps. Remember that it can continue to help. Try and use water cold enough to give yourself a good shock. Lastly, counting backwards or saying the alphabets backwards helps. It can start hard in the beginning and later you will find yourself saying the complete alphabets backwards.

"There are wounds that never show on the body that are deeper and more hurtful than anything that bleeds."
--Laurell K. Hamilton--

GROUND YOURSELF

Bring yourself mentally back to the present by grounding yourself. Experts believe, if you have suffered any kind of trauma, chances are that some things, such as specific smells, tastes, touches, or something someone says or does can trigger you. In an instant, you find yourself mentally transported back to the traumatic event. Flashbacks are scary, but there are some things you can do to help yourself mentally come back to the present. Here are some of the best grounding techniques doctors suggest. Please note, however, that not every grounding technique may work for you. Try different techniques to discover which ones work best for you specifically. Grounding techniques are those that help you focus on the here and now and remind you that you are not in the past traumatic experience. For example, listen to your favorite type of music. Concentrate on the lyrics and it may help to sing along with the lyrics as well.

Also, you can touch the things in your surroundings and name each thing as you touch it either in your head or aloud. It's been said doing so will help you concentrate on your current circumstances and reminds you that you are not in the past.

In addition, using repetitive phrases can help. Sometimes, repeating certain phrases will help you come back to the present. You might tell yourself, "I am safe now" or, "That Was then, this is now. "Keep repeating these phrases until you feel better you can talk or write it out. If someone is with you, and you can trust that person, talk to him or her about what you are feeling. Call a trusted friend and talk to him or her about what you are experiencing. Alternatively, call your therapist to talk and if no one is available, try writing down how you feel and what you are experiencing. Remind yourself that while you feel you are in the past traumatic experience, you are safe now. Also, pets are a wonderful way you can ground yourself. Just by brushing, petting, or play with your dog or cat if you have one. Animals can be extremely therapeutic. Even being near your pet may help you feel better. Read is another way to ground yourself. When you read, you must focus on the here and now. Read a book you enjoy. Do not read something that may remind you of the past trauma or could make you upset.

Finally, breathe properly by breathing with your diaphragm, in through your nose, and out through your mouth. Take several deep breaths using this method. Then, breathe in for two seconds, hold it for two seconds, breathe out for two seconds, and wait for two seconds. Repeat this several times. The counting in this technique will help you focus on the present as well as using visualization techniques to help calm your anxiety.

"That's the thing about depression: A human being can survive almost anything, as long as she sees the end in sight. But depression is a insidious, and it compounds daily, that it's impossible to ever see the end."
--Elizabeth Wurtzel--

GROUNDING TECHNIQUES

Experts believe grounding is a particular way of coping that is designed to "ground" you in the present moment. In doing so, you can retain your connection with the present moment and reduce the likelihood that you slip into a flashback or dissociation. In this way, grounding may be considered to be very similar to mindfulness. To ground, you want to use the five senses (sound, touch, smell, taste, and sight). To connect with the here and now, you want to do something that will bring all your attention to the present moment. In sum, here is a couple of grounding techniques doctors suggested described below.

1. **Sound:** Turn on loud music. Loud, jarring music will be hard to ignore. And as a result, your attention will be directed to that noise, bringing you into the present moment.

2. **Touch:** Grip a piece of ice. If you notice that you are slipping into a flashback or a dissociative state, hold onto a piece of ice. It will be difficult to direct your attention away from the extreme coldness of the ice, forcing you to stay in touch with the present moment.

3. **Smell:** Sniff some strong peppermint. When you smell something strong, it is very hard to focus on anything else. In this way, smelling peppermint can bring you into the present moment, slowing down or stopping altogether a flashback or an episode of dissociation.

4. **Taste:** Bite into a lemon. The sourness of a lemon and the strong sensation it produces in your mouth when you bite into the lemon it can force you to stay in the present moment.

5. **Sight:** Take an inventory of everything around you. Connect with the present moment by listing everything around you. Identify all the colors you see. Count all the pieces of furniture around you. List off all the noises you hear. Taking an inventory of your immediate environment can directly connect you with the present moment.

"You may not always have a comfortable life and you will not always be able to solve all of the world's problems at once but don't ever underestimate the importance you can have because history has shown us that courage can be contagious and hope can take on a life of its own."

--Michelle Obama—

MINDFULNESS

According to counseling professionals, mindfulness is the practice of purposely focusing your attention on the present moment and accepting it without judgment. Mindfulness is now being examined scientifically and has been found to be a key element in happiness. In recent years, psychotherapists have turned to mindfulness meditation as an important element in the treatment of a number of problems, including; depression, substance abuse, eating disorders, couples conflicts, anxiety disorders, and obsessive-compulsive disorder.

Some experts believe that mindfulness works by helping people to accept their experiences including painful emotions rather than react to them with hate and avoidance. It's become increasingly common for mindfulness meditation to be combined with psychotherapy, especially cognitive behavioral therapy. This development makes good sense, since both meditation and cognitive behavioral therapy share the common goal of helping people gain prospective on irrational, maladaptive, and self-defeating thoughts. It been said there is more than one way to practice mindfulness, but the goal of any mindfulness technique is to achieve a state of alert, focused relaxation by deliberately paying attention to thoughts and sensations without judgment. This allows the mind to refocus on the present moment. All mindfulness techniques are a form of meditation.

In addition, here are the basics of mindfulness meditation. First, sit quietly and focus on your natural breathing or on a word or "mantra" that you repeat silently. Allow thoughts to come and go without judgment and return to your focus on your breath or mantra. Second, focus on your body sensations; notice subtle body sensations such as an itch or tingling without judgment and let them pass. Notice each part of your body in succession from head to toe.

Third, you're sensory; notice sights, sounds, smells, tastes, and touches. Name the "sight," "sound," "smell," "taste," or "touch" without judgment and let them go. Firth, you're emotions. Allow emotions to be present without judgment. Practice a steady and relaxed naming of emotions: "joy," "anger," "frustration."

And, lastly, Urge surfing; cope with cravings (for addictive substances or behaviors) and allow them to pass. Notice how your body feels as the craving enters. Replace the wish for the craving to go away with the certain knowledge that it will subside.

"Three grand essentials to happiness in this life are something to do, something to love, and something to hope for."
--Joseph Addison--

KNOW YOUR TRIGGERS

Researchers discovered, triggers can be anything in your present day reality that reminds you either consciously or unconsciously, of past abuse. Sometimes survivors can easily see how a trigger connects to the abuse. Other times the connections are less clear, and survivors may know only that something bothers and upsets them. It's been said, memory loss is a frequent repercussion of abuse, and can keep survivors from understanding the reasons behind their reactions to certain situations. Some triggers may be difficult to identify because they are related to a highly specific aspect of the abuse. Since triggers can be almost anything, it is important to take seriously a person's reaction. Having awareness of triggers can give a person an insight into particulars about the abuse and help facilitate recovery. Identifying triggers gives the survivors power. Triggers lose their mystery and possibly their potency once they are understood. Once the mystery is explained, a person may still react, but may not be surprised or horrified by the reaction.

In addition, in coping with flashbacks and dissociation, prevention is the key. Research shows, flashbacks and dissociation are often triggered or cued by some kind of reminder of a traumatic event (for example, encountering certain people, going to specific places), or some other stressful experience. Therefore, it is important to identify the specific things that trigger flashbacks or dissociation. By knowing what your triggers are, you can either try to limit your exposure to those triggers, or if that is not possible (which is often the case), you can prepare for them by devising ways to cope with your reaction to those triggers.

Also, reducing flashbacks and dissociation, knowing your triggers may also help with other symptoms of PTSD, such as intrusive thoughts and memories of a traumatic event.

And, as soon as you notice that you are emotionally reacting, you have to shift your emotional state in order to think through what your trigger might be. Therefore, doctor's suggesting to practice the following: **Relax,** breathe and release the tension in your body; **Detach,** clear your mind of all thoughts; **Center,** drop your awareness to the center of your body just below your navel. Feel yourself breathe. This helps to clear the mind. And, focus, choose one keyword that represents how you want to feel or who you want to be in this moment. Once you shift your emotional state, you are free to examine if someone is actually taking something away from you or not. You can then ask for what you need or let it go and move on. Keep breathing and thinking of your keyword and you will be able to outsmart your brain.

"We have always held to hope, the belief, the conviction that there is a better life, a better world, beyond the horizon."
--Franklin D. Roosevelt--

IDENTIFY EARLY WARNING SIGNS

Symptoms do not usually just pop up out of the blue. They are usually preceded by some warning signs. These can be many (sometimes minor) things, such as the experience of certain emotions, changes in thoughts, or changes in behavior. Below are three common warning signs and examples that will help you identify your symptoms says counseling professionals.

First, you would notice changes in how you think for example, "I don't care about going to therapy anymore." Nothing is working out for me. I am never going to get better. No one cares about me or what I do. What's the point of going on? I'm feeling a little down. This must mean that I am going to fall into a deep depression again.

Second, you would notice changes in your mood for example, "everyone is getting on my nerves lately." I just don't feel happy, even when I am around people that I know I love. I am beginning to feel really jumpy and on edge. My mood keeps changing rapidly. In minutes, I can go from feeling really happy to really down or terrified.

Third, you would notice changes in your behavior: I just don't have the energy to take care of myself in the morning. "I haven't showered for days." I don't want to be around people anymore. "I've been isolating myself." I've been drinking more, but just to take the edge off of my feelings a little. I've notice that I am less talkative than I used to be."

In addition awareness of your own personal warning signs may make a return of PTSD symptoms feel more predictable and less unexpected. Recognition of your own warning signs also provides you with the opportunity to cope with these changes before they become unmanageable.

Once you have identified your warning signs, come up with a plan of action. You can turn to a therapist to help you with this, as well, Figure out how you can best cope. In addition, share you warning signs with a love one so that he/she can also be on the lookout and help you cope.

Also, flashbacks and dissociation may feel as though they come "out-of-the-blue." That is, they may feel unpredictable and uncontrollable. However, doctors believe there are often some early signs that a person may be slipping into a flashback or a dissociative state. For example, a person's surroundings may begin to look "fuzzy," or someone may feel as though he is separating from or losing touch with his surroundings, other people, or even himself.

> *"Flashbacks and dissociation are easier to cope with and prevent if you can catch them early on. Therefore, it is important to try to increase your awareness of early symptoms of flashbacks and dissociation. Next time you experience a flashback or dissociation, revisit what you were feeling and thinking just before the flashback or dissociation occurred. Try to identify as many early symptoms as possible. The more early warning signs you can come up with, the better able you will be to prevent future flashbacks or episodes of dissociation"*

> *"Hope is a waking dream."*
>
> *--Aristotle--*

US ALL YOUR SENSES

It's been suggested to us all your senses when trying to reduce flashbacks. Such as sound; blast yourself out of your pants. Loud, obnoxious music will be hard to ignore; it will keep you out of your head and grounded to the present moment. Also use your sense of touch; freeze you balls off, we all have that family member or friend that dumps ice down your back, remember how shocking it is? It's impossible to ignore right? That is the point, and although it may not be the most flattering method, there is no way you can ignore ice on you testicles. Sorry ladies, I can't say if it will have the same effect for you (smile). If you don't remember all your senses, just remember what you were taught in elementary school. Remember the sense of smell. Try your nostrils, scent is a powerful sense, if you overwhelm it with a strong scent it will keep you in the present. Heard of smelling salt? They can wake up someone who has gone unconscious just by how powerful the scent is. I don't really recommend using smelling salt, a method a little less harsh on the nostrils would be to smell some strong peppermint or putting your face into a jar of Vick's Vapor Rub that should do the trick.

In addition, let's not forget our sense of taste. Pucker up; ever had something so sour it made your whole face pucker? How likely would you be able to ignore something like that? Not very likely so if you catch an early warning sign and there's not a whole lot at your disposal and you see lemon, well, grab that little yellow devil and take a big bite. Your mind won't be focused on anything other than how incredibly sour that lemon is, episode averted.

Lastly, sight, you should take inventory of every item around you and of every sound you hear, but that's a bit too boring for me. It's time to go back to the days of when you were 13 (in Jr. High School) and you first found your dad's stash of magazines under the bed, the only thing that could break your concentration from those pages was the footsteps of your parents impending approach. Grab a magazine and get absorbed into taking inventory of everything you see in there, you get to avoid a flashback or dissociation and have a good time doing it. There is a lot of evidence showing these methods will help you reduce and prevent your flashbacks or dissociation, but I highly recommend seeking professional help as well.

> *"You can make positive deposits in your own economy every day by reading and listening to powerful, positive, life-changing content and by associating with encouraging and hope-building people."*
>
> --Zig Ziglar--

SELF-TALK

Over time, of course, giving yourself instructions becomes unnecessary for self talk, but while you're learning, it does three important things. First, it enhances our attention, focusing us on the important elements of the task and screening out distractions. Second, it helps us regulate our effort and make decisions about what to do, how to do it, and when. Third, self talk allows us to control our cognitive and emotional reactions, steadying us so we stay on task.

In a recent study of students learning to throw darts in a gym class; it was found most people don't realize it, but as we go about our daily lives we are constantly thinking about and interpreting the situations we find ourselves in. It's as though we have and internal voice inside our head that determines how we perceive every situation. Psychologist call this inner voice "self-talk", and it includes our conscious thoughts as well as our unconscious assumptions or beliefs. Most of our self-talk is reasonable, 'I'd better do some preparation for that exam", or 'I'm really looking forward to that match'. However, some of our self-talk is negative unrealistic or self-defeating, 'I'm going to fail for sure', or 'I didn't play well, I'm hopeless'.

In addition, self-talk is often slanted towards the negative, and sometimes it's just plain wrong. If you are experiencing depression, it is particularly likely that you interpret things negatively. That's why it's useful to keep an eye on the things you tell yourself, and challenge some of the negative aspects of your thinking. You can test, challenge and change your self-talk. You can change some of the negative aspects of your thinking by challenging the irrational parts and replacing them with more reasonable thoughts. With practice, you can learn to notice your own negative self-talk as it happens, and consciously choose to think about the situation in a more realistic and helpful way.

Lastly, the more you work on improving your self-talk the better you will get. It's kind of like practicing an instrument or going to sports training, it won't be easy to start with but will get better with time. It might not seem like much, but self-talk is a really important part of our self-esteem and confidence. By working on getting more positive self-talk, you're self-esteem and confidence, you are more likely to get things done and feel more in control of stuff that's going on in your life.

"We are only as strong as we are united, as weak as we are divided."

--J.K. Rowling--

DISPUTE NEGATIVE THOUGHTS

Psychologist says disputing your self-talk means challenging the negative or unhelpful aspects. Doing this enables you to feel better and to respond to situations in a more helpful way. Learning to dispute negative thoughts might take time and practice, but is worth the effort. Once you start looking at it, you'll probably be surprised by how much of your thinking is inaccurate, exaggerated, or focused on the negatives of the situation.

And, whenever you find yourself feeling depressed, angry, anxious or upset, use this as your signal to stop and become aware of your thoughts. Use your feelings as your cue to reflect on your thinking. A good way to test the accuracy of your perceptions might be to ask yourself some challenging question. It's been said these questions will help you to check out your self-talk to see whether your current view is reasonable. This will also help you discover other ways of thinking about your situation. Experts believe, these are the main types of challenging questions to ask yourself when checking your self-talk:

1. Reality testing
What is my evidence for and against my thinking?
Are my thoughts factual, or are they just my interpretations?
Am I jumping to negative conclusions?
How can I find out if my thoughts are actually true?

2. Look for alternative explanations
Are there any other ways that I could look at this situation?
What else could this mean?
If I were being positive, how would I perceive this situation?

3. Putting it in perspective

Is this situation as bad as I am making out to be?
What is the worst thing that could happen? How likely is it?
What is the best thing that could happen?
What is most likely to happen?
Is there anything good about this situation?
Will this matter in five years time?

When you feel anxious, depressed or stressed-out your self-talk is likely to become extreme, you'll be more likely to expect the worst and focus on the most negative aspects of your situation. So, it's helpful to try and put things into their proper perspective.

"Hope lies in dreams, in imagination, and in the courage of those who dare to make dreams into reality."
--Jonas Salk--

PEOPLE IN HISTORY AND MODERN TIMES WHO ACHIEVED GREAT THINGS

- **Buzz Aldrin**, one of America's most famous astronauts, flew to the moon in 1969, but later suffered from depression and alcoholism. He worked his way through, and even served as chairman of the National Mental Health Association.

- Performer **Adom Ant** says he has had a "lifelong battle against manic depression, "He has also been hospitalized for treatment of bipolar disorder.

- Comedienne **Roseanne Barr** has used antidepressants and psychotherapy after being diagnosed with depression in 1994.

- **Ludwig van Beethoven** experienced bipolar disorder, as documented in the book "The Key to Genius: Manic Depression and the Creative Life."

- Former Pittsburgh Steelers quarterback **Terry Bradshaw** was diagnosed with clinical depression and began taking antidepressants in the late 90s.

- Actor **Marlo Brando** experienced chronic depression throughout his life.

- Designing Women actress **Delta Burke** called her struggle with depression "lifelong" and said even as a teen she had trouble.

- **Earl Campbell**, former football pro and current business owner documented his personal struggle in

"The Earl Campbell Story: A Football Great's Battle with Panic Disorder."

- **Drew Carey** said he suffered through a long depression and at 18 and again in his 20s, attempted suicide with drug overdoses.

- **Jim Carrey** openly discussed his history of depression and being on Prozac on "60 Minutes" in 2004.

- Anthony Storr wrote about **Winston Churchill's** bipolar disorder in "Churchill's Black Dog, Kafka's Mine, and Other Phenomena of the Human Mind."

- **Dick Clark** talked about his experience with depression in the book, "On the Edge of Darkness" by Kathy Cronkite.

- Musician **Kurt Cobain** was diagnosed with attention deficit disorder at a young age and then later, with bipolar disorder.

- Singer **Judy Collins** suffered with depression, bulimia and alcoholism, particularly after her son committed suicide.
- SC author **Pat Conroy** battled depression his whole life and suffered a setback whe his schizophrenic brother committed suicide.

- **Calvin Coolidge**, thirtieth President of the United States, fell into a deep depression after the death of his son.

- In the late 1980s, singer **Sheryl Crow** had a period of depression after touring with Michael Jackson. Her depression was helped by antidepressants and therapy.

- **Golfer John Daly** admitted to depression and bouts of heavy drinking in interviews and the book "My Life in and Out of the Rough."

- **Diana, Princess of Wales** lived with bulimia and experienced bouts of depression.

- **Charles Dickens** depression was documented in the book "Key to Genius."

- Academy Award-winning actress patty Duke wrote about her bipolar disorder in two autobiographies.

- Famous for her role as Princess Leia in Star Wars, **Carrie Fisher** has lived with Bipolar Disorder for two decade and is severely manic depressive.

- **Al Gore's** estranged wife, tipper, experienced depression after her son's near fatal car accident in 1989. She was officially diagnosed with clinical depression two years later and fully recovered with medication and therapy.

- Terminator star **Linda Hamilton** has talked opening about a lifelong struggle with manic depression that went undiagnosed for most of her life.

- Pulitzer Prize-winning novelist **Ernest Hemingway's** suicidal depression is examined in the blood: "An Intimate Portrait of Ernest Hemingway by Those Who Knew Him" by Denis Brian.

- Singer **Janet Jackson** has chronically suffered from depression, especially for the two years preceding the release of "velvet rope."

- In the 1970s singer **Bill Joel** experienced serious depression and admitted himself into a hospital for treatment after a suicide attempt.

- **Catherine Zeta Jones'** rep said that the movie star checked into a facility for treatment of bipolar II disorder.

- Actress **Ashley Judd** has reveled that she had suffered from depression and an eating disorder.
- **Margot Kidder** who played Lois Lane in Superman says a combination of traditional and alternative medicine helped her overcome life-long depression.

- Prior to his death, "Brokeback Mountain" and "Dark Prince" star **Health Ledger** battled insomina, drug abuse and depression.

- Gone with the wind star **Vivien Leigh** suffered from mental illness, as documented in "Vivien Leigh: A Biography' by Ann Edwards.

- **President Abraham Lincoln's** first major depression happen in his 20s and he struggled with it for the remainder of his life, in addition to anxiety attacks.

- Olympic medal winning diver **Greg Louganis** first experience depression when he was 12 and he later attempted suicide twice.

- The mental illness of **Michelangelo** (dj Lodovico Buonarroti Simon), one of the greatest artistic geniuses in history, is discussed in "the Dynamics of Creation" by Anthony Storr.

- Scientist **Isaac Newton's** mental illness is a subject in "the Dynamics of Creation" by Anthony Storr and "the Key to Genius: Manic Depression and the Creative Life" by D. Jablow Hershman and Julian Lieb.

- Comedienne **Rosie O'Donnell** says her depression started to improve when she was 37 and began taking medication.

- **Marie Osmond** described a bout with postpartum depression in her book, "Behind the Smile."

- Former host of the Today Show and Dateline NBC **Jane Pauley** has been outspoken about living with bipolar disorder and depression

- Depression hit author, **J.K. Rowling** after her first marriage broke down after just two years. She credits writing her first Harry Potter novel with helping her overcome the depression.

- Actress **Winona Ryder** says she had panic attacks starting at 12 and ended up in a psychiatric clinic at 19 for treatment of severe depression.

- Actress **Brooke Shields** suffered from post-partum depression after the birth of her son.

- **Darryl Strawberry**, former baseball player for the New York Mets and the New York Yankees, reportedly has bipolar disorder.

- In an interview with the Daily Telegraph, Actress **Emma Thompson** said she battled clinical depression in the past, with her career saving her from "going under."

- **Leo Tolstoy**, author of "War and Peace," started experiencing depression while writing "Anna Karenina."

- Martial arts actor **John Claude Van Damme** started experiencing depression as a teen, but was not diagnosed with rapid cycling bipolar disorder until the late 90s.

- **Vincent Van Gogh's** bipolar disorder is also covered in "The Dey to Genius: Manic Depression and the Creative Life."

- 60 Minutes legend **Mike Wallace** was diagnosed with clinical depression in 1984 (after being sued for libel). He experienced severe depressive episodes, but overcame them with therapy and antidepressant medication.

- Heisman trophy winner **Ricky Williams** was diagnosed with social anxiety disorder.

- Country Music Hall of Fame country singer **Tammy Wynette** received electro-convulsive therapy for her depression.

Retrieve from Boston's News Leader (WCVB-TV)

http://therapist2013.wix.com/e-therapy

JUICE RECIPES FOR A HEALTHIER MENTAL HEALTH

Berry A-Peeling

Ingredients

- Apples - 2 large (3-1/4" dia) 446g
- Lime - 1/2 fruit (2" dia) 33.5g
- Strawberries - 3 cup, whole 432g
- 16oz

Directions

Process all ingredients in a juicer, shake or stir and serve.

*It has been shown that, besides having an anti-anemic effect, folic acid found in strawberries can help improve memory, concentration and the brain's ability to process information.

> "When you don't feel well, stop eating and go to juices."

> "Juices are like a blood transfusion. A glass of fruit and vegetable juice takes very little digestion, if any. It goes right into your body. We look at juices in the same way a doctor would look at an I.V It's something that can go right into your bloodstream."
> -- Dr. Richard Schulze : Juice-Fasting--

Minty Berry

Ingredients

- Blueberries - 2 cup 296g
- Kiwifruit - 2 fruit (2" dia) 138g
- Peppermint - 30 leaves 1.5g
- Strawberry - 1 cup, whole 144g
- 16oz

Directions

You may have issues juicing the mint leaves if you use a centrifuge juicer. Try to bunch them up into a tight ball or pack them into some lettuce before juicing. If all else fails, just stick a few mint leaves in the juice itself to get some of the minty flavor.

*It has been shown that, besides having an anti-anemic effect, folic acid found in strawberries can help improve memory, concentration and the brain's ability to process information. The high magnesium content in kiwifruit enhances energy production within the brain, thereby increasing concentration, memory, and relieving mental fatigue.

"Every day, give yourself a good mental shampoo."
                                              --Dr. Sara Jordan--

Fruity Punch with a Twist

Ingredients

- Apples - 2 medium (3" dia) 364g
- Kiwifruit - 4 fruit (2" dia) 276g
- Lemon (with rind) - 1/4 fruit (2-3/8" dia) 21g
- Lime (with rind) - 1/4 fruit (2" dia) 16.75g
- Oranges (peeled) - 2 fruit (2-5/8" dia) 262g
- Pineapple - 1 fruit 905g
- 16oz

Directions

Process all ingredients in a juicer, shake or stir and serve.

*The high magnesium content in kiwifruit enhances energy production within the brain, thereby increasing concentration, memory, and relieving mental fatigue.

"The greatest medicine of all is to teach people how not to need it."
--The Juice Master--

Red Dawn

Ingredients

- Apples - 2 medium (3" dia) 364g
- Cabbage (red) - 2 leaf 46g
- Carrots - 3 medium 183g
- Cucumber - 1 cucumber (8-1/4") 301g
- Mango (peeled) - 1 fruit without refuse 336g
- Strawberries - 1.5 cup, whole 216g
- 32oz

Directions

It has been shown that, besides having an anti-anemic effect, folic acid found in strawberries can help improve memory, concentration and the brain's ability to process information Process all ingredients in a juicer, shake or stir and serve.

*It has been shown that, besides having an anti-anemic effect, folic acid found in strawberries can help improve memory, concentration and the brain's ability to process information.

"If a drug company finds out that celery juice lowers blood pressure and if they tell it to people, they can't sell their drugs. They get three bucks for a pill. Why should they tell you to use celery juice?"
--Jacque Fresco--

http://therapist2013.wix.com/e-therapy

Appleberry Lush

Ingredients

- Apple - 1 medium (3" dia) 182g
- Carrots - 7 medium 427g
- Strawberry (heaping) - 1 cup, whole 144g
- 16oz

Directions

Process all ingredients in a juicer, shake or stir and serve.

*It has been shown that, besides having an anti-anemic effect, folic acid found in strawberries can help improve memory, concentration and the brain's ability to process information.

"Raw food expert Karen Knowler once wrote, fruit juices are good for picking you up. Vegetable juices make you feel truly nourished, and green juices balance you and help to reduce food cravings."
--Running on Juice--

Strawberry Mint Julep
This refreshing juice is extra delicious when made with white tea!

Ingredients

- Apples - 2 large (3-1/4" dia) 446g
- Green Tea - 1 cup 245g
- Honey (optional) - 1 tsp 7g
- Lemon - 1/4 fruit (2-1/8" dia) 14.5g
- Peppermint - 12 leaves 0.6g
- Strawberries - 1.5 cup, whole 216g
- 22oz

Directions
Steep a cup of green (or white) tea, and let cool.
Juice produce and herbs.
Pour cooled tea into juice, stir in honey, and serve over ice.

*It has been shown that, besides having an anti-anemic effect, folic acid found in strawberries can help improve memory, concentration and the brain's ability to process information.

"Sometimes you win, sometimes you learn."
--Anonymous--

Strawberry-Pineapple-Mint

Ingredients

- Pear - 1 medium 178g
- Peppermint - 15 leaves 0.75g
- Pineapple - 1/2 fruit 452.5g
- Strawberry - 1 cup, whole 144g
- 16oz

Directions

You may have issues juicing the mint leaves if you use a centrifuge juicer. Try to bunch them up into a tight ball or pack them into some lettuce before juicing. If all else fails, just stick a few mint leaves in the juice itself to get some of the minty flavor.

*It has been shown that, besides having an anti-anemic effect, folic acid found in strawberries can help improve memory, concentration and the brain's ability to process information.

"Make it happen today, and keep it moving."
--Patricia A. Carlisle--

Blackberry Pop

Ingredients

- Blackberry - 1 cup 144g
- Kiwifruit - 1 fruit (2" dia) 68g
- Pear - 1 medium 178g
- Peppermint (optional) - 10 leaves 0.5g
- Pineapple (peeled, cored) - 1/4 fruit 226.25g
- 16oz

Directions

Process all ingredients in a juicer, shake or stir and serve.

*The high magnesium content in kiwifruit enhances energy production within the brain, thereby increasing concentration, memory, and relieving mental fatigue.

"The body has what my father called; its own healing mechanism and he went further and said, "It's the doctor's duty to activate and reactivate the body's own healing mechanism."
--Charlotte Gerson from Food Matters—

HERBAL TEA FOR MENTAL HEALTH RECOVERY
TOP 10 RECIPES!

There are many medications that are designed for combating the symptoms of depression, along with anxiety and mood related emotions. Many of them come with side effects that some people find unwanted, and for some, depression is not an all the time occurrence. It may occur seasonally or in spurts instead. For these individuals, an herbal tea for depression may be just what the doctor ordered. There are many things that are found in nature that can help lift the spirits and counteract a down and out mood. Some of them have been extensively studied, and others simply hold a place in ancient medicine for bringing about feelings of happiness and joy. In spite of, some of the most powerful herbal remedies nature has to offer can help reverse a depressive state and combat anxiety, worry and stress as well.

Expert herbalist has compiled a list of the top ten herbs useful in this purpose. They can be used in a standalone brewed beverage or combined in a wide variety of herbal tea recipes for both flavor and function.

1. St. John's Wort: One of the most thoroughly studied herbs found in nature is St. John's Wort, which is also one of the most popular herbal remedies. It is available commercially and from health food stores and herbalist outlets. St. John's Wort is thought to balance out the chemicals in the brain that can affect mood, like serotonin, dopamine and norepinephrine. It also possesses antiviral and anti-inflammatory effects and is thought to support thyroid function too. Although easy to find in pill and supplement form, St. John's Wort lends itself nicely to brewing and can result in a delicious tea for depression that can lift the fog of a down and out mood.

2. Saffron: Saffron is best known for both its high price tag and its extensive use in exotic cuisine. But, saffron is much more than just a pricey flavoring. The spice is packed with vitamins, can help with digestive processes and also is thought to help boost a depressed mood. It goes without saying that it can make for a delicious tea for depression, boasting a unique and enjoyable flavor profile.

3. Rhodiola rosea: Rhodioloa rosea is a cold loving plant that has been used medicinally for a very long time. The plant has been associated with elevating the mood and affording the consumer a means to combat both stress and anxiety. Interestingly enough, the herb has also been linked to helping the bodies recover after physical activity, boosting immunity and improving mental acuity. Used in many herbal tea recipes and can be combined with other mood enhancing herbs into a unique and flavorful tea for depression symptoms.

4. Camu Camu: Camu Camu refers to a berry that grows in tropical regions and is thought to contain more vitamin C per serving than any other form of produce known. This herb is usually incorporated into blends based with green tea and it's thought to be able to combat the symptoms of depression with virtually no adverse side effects.

5. Maca: Maca is an interesting addition to our top ten lists because it has been studied extensively in one particular type of person – women experiencing the symptoms of menopause. Because mental changes occur commonly alongside the female change of life, the positive mental effects maca displayed in these studies was worth noting. Other studies showed that these same positive effects were observable in all individuals, not exclusive to those encountering menopause. Maca is an excellent addition to any tea for depression based on these results. Maca is available in many herbal tea blends, and the root is the part commonly used in these applications.

6. Ashwagandha: Ashwagandha is a plant that has been a mainstay of Ayurvedic medicine for a very long time. It has a wide range of medicinal benefits, including being an excellent addition to a tea for depression. This herb can help improve the mood and reduce anxiety as well. Ashwagandha also has shown some promise in terms of both cancer cell growth and degenerative diseases like Alzheimer's, making it arguably one of the most powerful herbs found in nature.

7. Rosemary: Best known for its role in culinary applications, rosemary also boasts a load of medicinal benefit that many people are unaware of. It is used in alternative medicine for bladder infections, diabetes and food poisoning but is thought to have another trick up its sleeve too. Rosemary is a notable addition to a tea for depression as the common kitchen herb is thought to help lift the spirits and reverse a depressed mood.

8. Passion Flower: Passion Flower is known for its sedative effects, and though that may not sound directly related to depression, the plant's ability to quell the stress and anxiousness that can accompany depression that make it an excellent choice. This herb is used for nerve disorders, muscle pain and emotional turmoil, all hallmark symptoms of depression. This herb is very popular in herbal tea recipes for its flavor and wide range of health benefits and makes an excellent addition to a tea for depression.

9. Chamomile: Much of what can cause or enhance the symptoms of depression centers around stress, worry and anxiousness. Chamomile, the herb that is well known for its use in helping people fall asleep, does a whole lot more than bring about a good night's rest. The reason why chamomile helps people to sleep is that it can reduce feelings of anxiety and provide a calming and relaxing sensation. For people who endure the symptoms of depression as they relate to anxiousness and worry, chamomile is an excellent choice.

10. Green Tea: Green tea is incredibly unique in that it actually promotes mental clarity while at the same time reducing the feelings of stress and anxiety that some people experience. It can lead to a truly focused state, which can be a great advantage for people battling the symptoms of depression. The beverage can serve as a tea for depression on its own, or combined with other herbs that can help to boost your mood and lift your spirits.

NOTE: Mental illness can be a serious medical condition and should be cared for by a trained medical provider. Persons with depression, especially those on medications, should not use alternative therapies without talking to their doctor beforehand. Herbal teas provide natural healing options without many of the risks associated with medications, and their safe and responsible use can lead to a reduction in the symptoms of depression and a relaxed and calm state without anxiousness, fear or worry.

RESOURCES

Holistic Measures. Comprehensive Behavioral Healthcare. http://therapist2013.wix.com.e-therapy 216-633-9858

Dharma Healing and Wellness, LLC. Life coaching, Law of Attraction Coaching, Relationship, Parent and Teen Life Coaching. http://www.dharmahw.com 216-551-3980

Holistic Online. http://www.holisticonline.com

American Music Therapy Association. Anger management and music therapy. http://www.musictherapy.org

International Guide to the World of Alternative Mental Health. Herbs for Treatment of Emotional and Mental States: by Gayle Eversole, DHom, PhD, RN (CP) http://alternativementalhealth.com

Happy Juicer. How diet affects mental health. http://www.happyjuicer.com

Adolescent Suicide Hotline, 1-800-621-4000

Adolescent Crisis Intervention & counseling Nineline. 1-800-999-9999

AIDS National Hotline. 1-800-432-2437

CHADD-Children & Adults with Attention Deficit/Hyperactivity disorder. 1-800-233-4050.

Child Abuse Hotline. 1-800-4-A-CHILD

Cocaine Helpline. 1-800-COCAINE (1-800-262-2463)

Domestic Violence Hotline. 1-800-799-7233

Domestic Violence Hotline/Child Abuse. 1-800-4-A-CHILD (1-800-422-4434)

Eating Disorders Center. 1-888-236-1188

Ecstasy Addiction. 1-800-468-6933

Family Violence Prevention Center. 1-800-313-1310

Gay & Lesbian national Hotline. 1-888-THE-GLNH (1-888-843-4564

Gay & Lesbian Trevor Helpline Suicide Prevention. 1-800-850-8075

Healing Women Foundation. (Abuse). 1-800-477-4111

Incest Awareness Foundation. 1-888-547-3222

Learning Disabilities-(National Center For). 1-888-575-7373

Missing & Exploited Children Hotline. 1-800-843-5678

National Alliance on Mental Illness (NAMI). 1-800-950-NAMI (6264)

Panic Disorder Information Hotline. 1-800-64-PANIC

Post Abortion Trauma. 1-800-593-2273

Project Inform HIV/AIDS Treatment Hotline. 1-800-822-7422

Rape (People Against Rape). 1-800-656-HOPE (1-800-656-4673)

Runaway Hotline. 1-800-621-4000

Self-Injury. (Information only) (Not a crisis line; Information and referrals only) 1-800-DONTCUT (1-800-366-8288)

Sexual Assault Hotline. 1-800-656-4673

Sexual Abuse-Stop It Now! 1-888-PREVENT

STD Hotline. 1-800-227-8922

Suicide Prevention Lifeline. 1-800-273-TALK

Suicide & Crisis Hotline 1-800-999-9999

Suicide Prevention-The Trevor Help Line. (Specializing in gay and lesbian youth suicide prevention) 1-800-850-8078

Teen Helpline. 1-800-400-0900

Victim Center. 1-800-FYI-CALL (1-800-394-2255)

Youth Crisis Hotline. 1-800-HIT-HOME

MESSAGE FROM THE AUTHOR

Most people who have mental health problems are often happy to pass on what they have learned from their experiences to others in the same situation. I spoke to people who were at different stages of their mental health recovery, and some were more hopeful than others about the future. Most of the people I interviewed were happy to discuss what help them in their recovery so it can inspire and give hope to other people with mental health problems, their families and in their careers. It was said, they knew what it was like to be diagnosis with a mental illness or to wake up and not feel "normal" every day. The techniques in this book was tried and proven by them and it was said it helped them with their symptoms. My message to you is … practice these techniques until you are able to claim them as your coping skills.

Remember, all is not lost there is life after a mental health diagnosis. I want you to know there is life after being diagnosed with a mentally illness, dealing with mental distress or, living within the mental health system. I would say, if you know you're behaving weirdly or if you've done something weird and you know there is something wrong; you will have to come to terms with that. And I think coming to terms with your mental illness is the biggest thing for people to do when they are suffering with the illness.

And, if something has gone wrong at some point in your life maybe not permanently wrong but something has gone wrong at some point. I think your first step is to come to terms with it and then be adventurous about what will heal you or get you better and get you back to some kind of "normal" state. As a professional therapist, I think you should try different things that you know can aid in your healing and listen to your inner self about what is good for you, you know, whether it's counseling or, if its therapy or a group session or whatever; just try and listen to yourself about what would be good for you; because if you don't someone else with make the decision for you, and I hope this book will help you make the right choice that will be best for you. Some people see their mental health problems as a kind of "enabling disability" But it can become a gift if you can learn to manage it. So although having a mental illness could change you forever, it might be a positive experience as well. I wish you peace and happiness in your spiritual journey.

www.ingramcontent.com/pod-product-compliance
Lightning Source LLC
Chambersburg PA
CBHW051623170526
45167CB00001B/35